CURING HEALTH CARE

Donald M. Berwick
A. Blanton Godfrey
Jane Roessner

with special contributions by
Paul E. Plsek
and
David A. Garvin

CURING HEALTH CARE

New Strategies
for Quality Improvement

A Report on the
National Demonstration Project on
Quality Improvement in Health Care

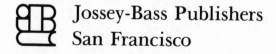 Jossey-Bass Publishers
San Francisco

CURING HEALTH CARE
New Strategies for Quality Improvement
by Donald M. Berwick, A. Blanton Godfrey, and Jane Roessner

Copyright © 1990 by: Jossey-Bass Inc., Publishers
350 Sansome Street
San Francisco, California 94104

Library of Congress Cataloging-in-Publication Data

Berwick, Donald M. (Donald Mark), date.
    Curing health care : new strategies for quality improvement /
Donald M. Berwick, A. Blanton Godfrey, Jane Roessner : with special
contributions by Paul E. Plsek and David A. Garvin.
       p.   cm. — (Jossey-Bass health series)
    Includes bibliographical references.
    Includes index.
    ISBN 1-55542-294-2
    1. Medical care — United States — Quality control.   2. Medical care —
United States — Evaluation.   I. Godfrey, A. Blanton.   II. Roessner,
Jane.   III. Title.   IV. Series.
    [DNLM: 1. Quality of Health Care — United States.   W 84 AA1 B45c]
RA399.A3B47   1990
362.1'0973 — dc20
DNLM/DLC
for Library of Congress   90-5229
                                                         CIP

Manufactured in the United States of America

 The paper used in this book is acid-free and meets the
State of California requirements for recycled paper
(50 percent recycled waste, including 10 percent
postconsumer waste), which are the strictest guidelines
for recycled paper currently in use in the United States.

JACKET DESIGN BY WILLI BAUM
FIRST EDITION

HB Printing   10 9 8 7

Code 9097

The Jossey-Bass Health Series

Contents

Foreword

It is common knowledge that health care has improved remarkably over the centuries. We live longer and healthier lives than our forebears, mainly because of advances in the numerous subsystems of the health industry, such as medical research, professional training for personnel, nutrition, and sanitation. To be sure, other industries also have made remarkable advances during those same centuries. Nevertheless, if a public poll were taken, the health industry would be widely acclaimed for its record of responsiveness to human needs.

However, this industry also faces severe criticism for alleged shortcomings: the rising price of health care, with no end in sight; the long periods of waiting for service; the allegedly high error rate; and even evidence of greed and fraud in some sectors of the industry.

Such real and imagined shortcomings have long existed in all industries and institutions, and to those institutions Darwin's concept of the survival of the fittest has universally applied. Institutions that responded to customer needs survived. Those that did not respond became extinct — replaced by competitors that provided society with better service and lower prices. Such competition for survival is now beginning to take place in the health industry. A variety of organizational forms are all trying to expand their share of the market by providing superior service and lower prices.

The key to successful competition lies in the concept of *fitness for survival*. When we transfer that concept from biological species to human institutions, we are dealing mainly with the interrelated parameters of quality and cost. During the last few decades, a number of our industrial institutions have strengthened their fitness by completing hundreds and even thousands of projects that have improved quality while at the same time reducing costs. The demonstration projects described in the present book establish publicly what has long been known to pioneering investigators: It is equally feasible to carry out quality improvement and cost reduction projects in the health industry.

These same demonstration projects also establish that the health industry now has a major opportunity to increase the pace of its improvements. Such progress cannot be made through more and more demonstration projects. Instead, it must be achieved by providing hospitals and other local institutions with the means for carrying out quality improvements on their own.

As the health industry undertakes this change, it is well advised to take into account the experience of other industries in order to understand what has worked and what has not. Of course, in the minds of many, the health industry is "different." This is certainly true as to its history, technology, and culture. However, the decisive factors in what works and what does not are the managerial processes, which are alike for all industries.

We can easily identify the success factors for those institutions that have already dramatically improved quality and reduced quality-related costs:

- The upper managers personally directed a new approach to managing for quality though creating and serving on a guiding quality council.
- They applied quality improvement methods to business processes as well as to traditional operating processes, and they attended to the needs of internal customers as well as to those of external customers.
- They adopted the concept of mandated, annual quality improvement. To this end they instituted an infrastructure to

identify needed improvements and to assign clear responsibility for making those improvements.

- They adopted the concept that planning for quality should involve participation by those who will be impacted by the plan.
- They adopted a modern quality-oriented methodology to replace empiricism in quality planning.
- They attempted to train all members of the hierarchy in the modern processes of managing for quality: quality planning, quality control, and quality improvement.
- They provided the work force with opportunities to receive training and to participate actively in the processes of managing for quality.
- The enlarged their strategic business plans to include quality goals and means for meeting those goals.

These are the most successful strategies to have evolved out of extensive experience in our industrial institutions. Institutions that have adopted these strategies have achieved enviable results. Other institutions that have opted for different strategies have far less to show for their effort and for the years that have elapsed.

The health industry faces similar options; it must choose its strategies carefully. Health industry managers are well advised to study carefully the lessons learned from the demonstration projects discussed in this book. Of these lessons, the most important involve the cause-and-effect relationships: Which managerial processes produced the results? Mastery of those managerial processes is the prerequisite for lasting success.

Wilton, Connecticut
August 1990

Joseph M. Juran
Chairman Emeritus
Juran Institute, Inc.

Preface

The paradox is infuriating. In some ways, it is the best of times for American health care. Medicine today deserves to boast about the power of its technologies, the depth of its bioscientific roots, the grandeur of its facilities, and the audacity of its reach into the human body. Cardiac surgeons repair infant heart defects that were inoperable and fatal a decade ago. Premature infants weighing barely a pound at birth survive and, in many cases, can look forward to normal lives. A leukemic five-year-old child has a 95 percent chance of cure; twenty years ago he or she would have had a 100 percent certainty of dying.

But in equally striking ways, it is the worst of times for American health care, at least since it entered the scientific era of twentieth-century practice. Almost no one is happy with the health care system. It costs too much; it excludes too many; it fails too often; and it knows too little about its own effectiveness. Mainly, though, it costs too much. Increasingly angry payers watched helplessly as America's health care costs doubled in the 1970s. Then, mocking the cost-containment efforts that followed, the costs doubled again in the 1980s.

The mood now of the physician, the patient, the administrator, and the payer alike is easy to label: *frustration*. The steps taken so far to control costs and improve the value of health care have not worked. Yet those leaders whose decisions will shape health care from now on seem lacking in fresh ideas. What can we possibly do to recapture control and hope in a system that feels so out of control and lacking in optimism about its future?

That, at bottom, is what this book is really about: recapturing hope. We think that there is at least one way out for American health care in the 1990s, namely, for health care organizations to learn and to apply the methods of modern quality management as their primary operating strategy. We base that belief on the evidence of extraordinary turnarounds in other industries in the past two decades, industries no less distressed or threatened in the past than American medicine is today. For those other industries, the threat was offshore — Japanese companies, mainly, that were deploying modern methods for the improvement of products and services and thereby achieving entirely unprecedented levels of efficiency and performance.

That story, and the story of American companies that woke up and began to use and benefit from quality management methods, has been told and retold in an excellent and growing literature on industrial quality improvement. Until now, however, no similar stories have been told about medical organizations. There have been no compelling health care examples. The reason is simple: Health care is a newcomer to modern quality improvement. The explanation for this is too complex for a preface; we will tackle it later on. But, in one sense, it does not matter why. It is, to put it bluntly, high time for health care to catch up.

This book reports on a beginning. The real story has been written by twenty-one health care organizations and an equal number of industrial quality management experts who first came together at a meeting in Boston in the fall of 1987 to launch what we have come to call the National Demonstration Project on Quality Improvement in Health Care — NDP for short. That project, funded by The John A. Hartford Foundation and hosted by the Harvard Community Health Plan, was an experiment designed to answer this question: *Can the tools of modern quality improvement, with which other industries have achieved breakthroughs in performance, help in health care as well?* The participant health care organizations, assisted by their assigned quality expert, formed teams to tackle this question locally in their own real-world operations through specific pilot projects. In June 1988, they reported back.

This book is an extended interpretation of their experiences — first steps toward an answer to the question, Can quality improvement help? We use their actual stories as a starting point for more theoretical discussions of the technology of quality improvement, but it is what they did that really matters.

Audience for the Book

We have written this book for several groups to use. First, we have in mind the managers and leaders of health care organizations — hospitals, health maintenance organizations, group practices, and nursing homes, for example — who, aware of both the current difficulties and the troubles yet to come, want to know more about how modern quality improvement methods might help them. We believe that the managers want specific case examples; they want to know what quality improvement would look like not just in theory but "on the ground."

Clinicians — even those without management roles — will be interested in thinking with us about the potential of these methods to improve clinical practice, an exciting area of application that several NDP project teams approached (though none as directly as we think possible in the future).

Those who pay for health care and those who regulate it may wish to identify and encourage health care suppliers who are truly serious about internal quality improvement efforts. This book may offer payers and regulators some concrete images of such efforts, so that they become more easily recognizable.

Those industrial companies that have made such giant strides in total quality management have shared their competence freely with many of their suppliers. They may wish to share similarly now with one of their most important suppliers — the health care organizations that take care of their employees.

Many excellent consultants in quality management, no matter how experienced in manufacturing issues, may yet regard medical care as forbidding territory for their badly needed skills. We intend this book to be helpful to them in translating ideas from manufacturing process improvement into medical images and medical settings.

We are also interested in contributing to the education of the students of medicine and management who will be the leaders of tomorrow's health care system. Until now, these students have lacked a book that serves as a teaching resource on quality improvement as a discipline specifically applied to medical settings. Similarly, organizations training their staffs in quality improvement can now rely on this book for useful case materials and graphic examples of health care applications.

Overview of the Contents

Chapter One explores the current state of the health care system and discusses the need for new methods of improvement. Chapter Two suggests the ways in which quality management can help meet the needs outlined in the first chapter. Chapter Three introduces the origins, theory, and vocabulary of modern industrial quality management. Chapters Four through Eight describe and analyze the specific experiences of the NDP teams as they worked their way through five basic steps in the quality improvement process on an issue each had selected in advance. We illustrate each step by drawing from and commenting on the actual project team reports. Chapter Nine is our own summary of lessons from the project, and the afterword, by David A. Garvin of the Harvard Business School, offers further summary reflections and conclusions.

Resource A is a roster of participants in the NDP. Resource B is a detailed discussion of quality improvement tools; it was written by a key adviser to the NDP, Paul E. Plsek, a statistical process control consultant who has become familiar with the needs and opportunities in health care. In Resource C, we present three actual team reports as representatives of the excellent work of all twenty-one participating health care organizations and their advisers.

The critical reader will notice that the strength of this book—its foundation in real projects in real organizations—is also its weakness. These teams actually existed; they actually struggled with the challenges of adapting these methods to health care and with the resistance to change that awaits any who begin the journey to quality improvement. They did take the first steps and proved that others can, too.

But because these are real stories, there are no astounding results to report. How could there be in a project that lasted only eight months? No hospital in these eight months turned around its bottom line. No team reaped million dollar successes. So far as we know, no single life was saved.

Before disappointment wins out, however, take a closer look. By different measures—the measures of new ways of thinking, new insights about work processes, new working relationships, and small, permanent breakthroughs in understanding—by these simple, modest measures of early success, the achievements of these pioneer project teams exceeded our most optimistic hopes. The glamour in what they did is not in the results achieved—those, we believe, will follow later as commitment and experience grow—but rather in the innovation begun. The first steps were taken by real organizations toward something truly new in an industry that desperately needs new ideas for helping itself.

Acknowledgments

We are grateful for the contributions of scores of people whose work has made this book possible. The members of the advisory committee for the National Demonstration Project—Paul Batalden, Howard Frazier, David Garvin, David Gustafson, David Hemenway, Marian Knapp, Ellen Marszalek-Gaucher, Lincoln Moses, Frederick Mosteller, Heather Palmer, Mitchell Rabkin, James Roberts, James Schlosser, and Debra Shenk—gave freely of their valuable time to guide and shape the project from its inception. The project participants—representatives of the health care organizations and the industrial quality experts—along with their sponsoring organizations were the true driving force behind the entire effort. It was inspiring to watch their enthusiasm, their openness, and their growing optimism as their work proceeded.

The work of the NDP and the production of this book have rested on the shoulders of a wonderful team of staff in the NDP itself, including Emily Bliss, Penny Carver, AnnMarie DeMarini, Joanne Healy, Judith Kalman, Richard Keene, Ellen McIntire, Ruth Manuel, James Schlosser, and Karen Schwartz. Jennifer Edwards of the Juran Institute also contributed much to the production of this book.

Many other organizations have contributed time and expertise to the project, including the Hospital Corporation of America, through its Quality Resource Group; the Juran Institute; and the host institution for the NDP, the Harvard Community Health Plan. Financial support has come generously from The John A. Hartford Foundation, whose officers Richard Sharpe and Mary Paulsen were unfailingly helpful, and from the Harvard Community Health Plan Foundation, whose executive director, Susan Pauker, was also a source of continuing encouragement. One of the leaders of current research on statistical methods in quality improvement, George Box, contributed an enlightening address at our planning conference. Rand Warren worked hard editing early versions of the project reports on which the book is based, and helpful criticisms were offered by Ann Berwick, John Early, Alain Enthoven, and John Ritchie. We are grateful to two giants in the quality field, Dr. Joseph M. Juran and Dr. Avedis Donabedian, who lent their visible support and ideas through their participation in the NDP Summative Conference.

Writing a book demands a great deal from the families of the authors. We want to acknowledge the tolerance, support, and encouragement we received from our families, especially when we were faced with the pressure of deadlines. Judith Godfrey; John Ritchie; Alexander and Rachel Roessner-Ritchie; Ann, Benjy, Daniel, Jessica, and Becca Berwick — thank you.

Finally, we would like to take special notice of the contribution of a single individual, Thomas O. Pyle, chief executive officer of the Harvard Community Health Plan, whose imagination lies at the base of the work reported here. His early suggestion that health care might well have something to learn by searching outside its own walls for ideas about quality, and his subsequent willingness to support and encourage that explora-tion, led directly to the collaboration that eventually matured into the NDP, this book, and the related activities that have grown and prospered since.

August 1990

Donald M. Berwick
Newton, Massachusetts

A. Blanton Godfrey
Wilton, Connecticut

Jane Roessner
Newton, Massachusetts

The Authors

Donald M. Berwick, M.D., has been a pediatrician at Harvard Community Health Plan since 1980 and served as vice president for quality-of-care measurement from 1985 to 1989. Dr. Berwick is a Phi Beta Kappa graduate of Harvard College, with an A.B. degree (1968), summa cum laude, in social relations. He received his M.A. degree (1972) in public policy from the John F. Kennedy School of Government at Harvard University. He received his M.D. degree (1972), cum laude, from the Harvard Medical School.

Dr. Berwick is a member of the faculty at the Harvard School of Public Health and associate professor of pediatrics at Harvard Medical School. He serves as a principal investigator for the National Demonstration Project on Quality Improvement in Health Care and is a judge for the Malcolm Baldrige National Quality Award. He is the author of numerous research papers on quality, decision analysis, technology assessment, and clinical evaluation.

From 1983 to 1985, he was associate director of the Institute for Health Research, a joint venture of Harvard University and Harvard Community Health Plan. He has been associate in pediatrics at Boston's Children's Hospital since 1978 and pediatrician at the Kenmore Center, Harvard Community Health Plan, since 1979. He is a past president of the Society for Medical Decision Making.

A. Blanton Godfrey has been chairman and CEO of Juran Institute, Inc., Wilton, Connecticut, since August 1987. He received his B.S. degree (1963) from Virginia Tech in physics. He received his M.S. (1970) and Ph.D. (1974) degrees from Florida State University in statistics.

Dr. Godfrey has been a member of the faculty of Columbia University since 1982, where he serves as an adjunct associate professor in the School of Engineering. He serves as a principal investigator for the National Demonstration Project on Quality Improvement in Health Care and is a judge for the Malcolm Baldrige National Quality Award. He is a fellow of the American Statistical Association, a fellow of the American Society for Quality Control, an academician of the International Academy for Quality, and a member of Sigma Xi. He is the author of numerous papers and chapters on quality improvement, quality management, and statistics. The previous book he coauthored, *Modern Methods for Quality Control and Improvement* (with Wadsworth and Stephens), was named Book of the Year by the Institute of Industrial Engineers in 1987.

From 1982 to 1987 he was head of the Quality Theory and Technology Department at AT&T Bell Laboratories. After joining Bell Labs in 1973, he was a member of the Technical Staff, supervisor of the Field Quality Theory and Systems Group, and head of the Network Performance Characterization Department.

Jane Roessner is a free-lance writer in the Boston area. She received her B.A. degree (1971) from Wellesley College in English and her Ph.D. degree (1976) from Boston College in English.

Since 1984, she has worked on a variety of free-lance writing projects, including scripts for multi-image, video, and planetarium productions, speeches, annual reports, and curriculum materials for such clients as WGBH, The Museum of Science, Massport, Children's Hospital, Hewlett-Packard, Converse, Wang, Polaroid, and Lotus. Her scholarly publications include "Double Exposure: Shakespeare's Sonnets 100–114" (*English Literary History,* Fall, 1979) and "The Coherence and the Context of Shakespeare's Sonnet 116" (*Journal of English and Germanic Philology,* July, 1982).

Dr. Roessner was an instructor of English at the University of Massachusetts, Boston, from 1976 to 1981, an assistant professor of English at Wellesley College from 1981 to 1982, and an assistant professor of English at the Massachusetts Institute of Technology from 1982 to 1984.

CURING HEALTH CARE

1

Symptoms of Stress in
the Health Care System

"She died, but she didn't have to."

The senior resident was sitting, near tears, in the drab office behind the nurses' station in the intensive care unit. It was 2:00 A.M., and he had been battling for thirty-two hours to save the life of the twenty-three-year-old graduate student who had just suffered her final cardiac arrest.

The resident slid a large manila envelope across the desktop. "Take a look at this," he said. "Routine screening chest X-ray, taken ten months ago. The tumor is right there, and it was curable — then. By the time the second film was taken eight months later, because she was complaining of pain, it was too late. The tumor had spread everywhere, and the odds were hopelessly against her. Everything we've done since then has really just been wishful thinking. We missed our chance. She missed her chance."

Exhausted, the resident put his head in his hands and cried.

Two months later, the Quality Assurance Committee completed its investigation. This death, like all others in this hospital, was reviewed in the biweekly meeting (6:00 to 8:00 P.M., every other Wednesday) of the group of five doctors and two nurses. They sat together over deli sandwiches, read records, and assigned the quality assurance nurse the job of tracking down

1

suspicious details and clearing up hazy facts. Their work was partially protected from legal discovery — an important detail in cases like this one, where a lawsuit was possible. Even so, the legal climate in this particular state was such that the hospital's attorney had advised the committee long ago to shred all notes except formal minutes and the carefully worded final report. That was standard operating procedure.

"We find the inpatient care commendable in this tragic case," concluded the brief report, "although the failure to recognize the tumor in a potentially curable stage ten months earlier was unfortunate. Despite this circumstance, the treating physicians used all proper procedures for treatment once the tumor was finally recognized."

Nowhere in the report was it written explicitly why the results of the first chest X-ray had not been translated into action. No one knew. At the time of readmission, a copy of the radiology report from that test had been located in the X-ray file room, and it clearly stated that the X-ray was suspicious: "Mediastinum widened; suspect possible mass lesion. Recommend tomography if clinically indicated." The internist who had ordered that X-ray had office notes reflecting the order: "Healthy twenty-two-year-old anthropology student. Slight cough. Exam normal in detail. Periods regular. Smokes ½ pack per day. Routine blood count and screening chest X-ray ordered." Yet no X-ray report was found in the doctor's office folder.

One year later, on the exact anniversary of the woman's death, the membership of the Quality Assurance Committee had changed completely. All members served on a voluntary basis for two years, and all the terms had expired. The senior resident had completed his training and had joined a group practice in Pittsburgh. The parents of the dead woman were at home sleeping, having completed plans for the unveiling of their daughter's gravestone.

It was 2:00 A.M., and the night custodian was cleaning the radiologist's office. As he moved a filing cabinet aside to sweep beneath it, he glimpsed a dusty tan envelope that had been stuck between the cabinet and the wall. The envelope contained a yellow radiology report slip, and the date on the report —

nearly two years earlier—convinced the custodian that this was, indeed, garbage. If it were important, he reasoned, it would have been missed or replaced by now. He tossed it in with the other trash, and four hours later it was incinerated along with other useless things.

Quality.   When the night custodian discarded the errant radiology report, he wrote the final page in a story of flaw. The defect, in this case, was fatal. Where did it come from? Who was responsible? It is easy to see quality in health care as a simple matter of people—doctors, usually—just doing their jobs right. According to that theory, quality is in the will and the skill of the people: their decisions, their competence, their motives.

But look deeper. Where did quality fail for the dying woman in our story? In the skill or the will of the radiologist who read the first film? In the motivation or thoroughness of the internist who ordered it routinely in a day filled with dozens of other routine events? Or was it in the radiology department manager who did not have the budget that year to set up a new computer tracking system for reports? Or in the secretary who never thought of setting up a log of reports awaiting signature? Or in the temporary secretary who, filling in on that particular day, did not happen to know about a logbook that, after all, *did* exist? Was it the people, or the equipment, or the rules, or the supplies? Or was it just an accident of fate that slid that envelope onto the floor when no one was watching? And, after all is said and done, will it happen again?

We want to believe in health care—in the trusted doctor, the chrome-clad hospital, the gentle touch. We need something to rely on—sources of help in our fear, our pain, or our dotage. We want to trust, and we expect excellence.

The profession of medicine wants, in its turn, to be trusted, and it, too, prizes excellence. Quality is implicitly guaranteed by the social contract between medicine and those it serves. Yet these are times of exceptional discomfort, both in medicine and in those who rely on it. The fabric of trust has worn thin. Pick up the Sunday newspaper and you will be less likely to discover a discussion of excellence in health care than an article spotlighting its vulnerability or failure. Pick up a medical trade journal and you will be less likely to find evidence of pride than of defense, fear, or uncertainty about the future. What has become of patients' confidence and physicians' pride? We are not celebrating the quality of health care today as much as we are questioning it. What has changed?

A Revolution in Accountability

In the 1990s, health care is experiencing a degree of change in its structure and relationship to society unparalleled at least since the influential *Flexner Report* of the early 1900s ushered medicine into its era of scientific training and away from the apprenticeships that characterized medical education in the late nineteenth century. Before Flexner, physicians were initiates into a brotherhood passing on the wisdom of its elders; after Flexner, physicians were applied scientists, seeking rationale in scientific theory. In both eras, however, they were members of a profession in full command of the right to judge the quality of what they did, and, as it happened, in nearly full command of the economic rules under which they did their work.

As the twentieth century ends, health care is undergoing a second revolution: not a revolution in theory, but a revolution in the locus of control. One hundred years ago, power was about to shift in substantial measure away from practitioners and toward medical scientists, but the shift occurred *within* the profession. Doctors won power from doctors. The modern shift cuts far more fundamentally into the profession from the outside; it is a wresting of significant amounts of control from the profession by others outside the profession.

The modern revolution is a revolution in *accountability*. Practitioners used to justify their clinical choices, if at all, only to each other, and only informally. Today, managed care systems, government agencies, utilization review departments, and payers are scrutinizing care, and with decreasing reluctance asking doctors and hospitals to explain what they do and why they do it. Doctors and hospitals used to be able to count on *someone* paying for whatever they chose to do. No longer. Prepaid care systems, government regulation, and price competition are gradually replacing "cost-plus" health care reimbursement. Standards, protocols, and guidelines are bearing down on "professional autonomy," and doctors loudly bemoan the threat of "cookbook medicine," by which they mean the prescription *to them* of the diagnostic and treatment strategies they will be permitted to use and for which they will be paid.

Why the Change?

Cost, more than anything else, is driving the change. Look at it from the point of view of the main payer for health care in this country: the American corporation.

In 1987, American automobile manufacturers were deep into a struggle for survival in a worldwide marketplace. The hegemony of American manufacturing was only a memory. Competitive advantage was to be won, not assumed. The chief executive officer of the American automobile company knew that every car rolling off the assembly line in Detroit contained, in the insurance premiums for health care paid by the employer for the employees, $700 worth of health care. Blue Cross had become, in effect, the car companies' biggest supplier. In aggregate, the 1989 health care bill for the United States was over $600 billion, more than 11 percent of the gross national product. This was so large a sum that, if the American health care industry were declared a nation, it would have the sixth largest GNP of all the nations on earth.

The gargantuan health care bill has been a problem on the national agenda at least since the early 1970s, when a worried government and frightened payers undertook a series of initiatives intended to control the rate of increase of that bill, which has historically grown far faster than the cost of living. Government, which pays for 40 percent of American health care, introduced various experiments based on differing theories of why costs grew so fast and how they could best be contained:

- *Foster Competition.* Change regulations and payment procedures to allow health care providers to bid against each other for market share. Let market forces drive prices down.

- *Limit the Total Payment.* Declare unwillingness to pay more than a certain total amount for health care, and hold hospitals to these bottom lines, using the force of regulation and the power of the checkbook.
- *Limit Unit Prices.* Define clusters of disease or episodes of care, and notify providers in advance that they will be paid only a certain, fixed amount for the care of a patient in that condition. Beyond that cost, the provider — not the payer — absorbs the financial risk.
- *Encourage Better Management of Care.* On the theory that waste abounds, create financial incentives to encourage efficiencies instead of letting inefficient producers of care simply pass their unnecessary costs through to consumers. The main mechanism used to encourage efficiency has been prepayment — that is, paying providers "up front" for the care of defined populations, giving the provider a stake in parsimony. The health maintenance organization, in which the insurance function and the care-giving function merge, is the most important form of such prepaid, managed care.
- *Limit the Definition of "Health Care" Itself.* Trim the insurance benefit by excluding population subgroups (for example, those with bad health histories) from coverage, or by deciding that certain services (for example, marital counseling, or cosmetic surgery, or procedures of uncertain benefit) will not be called "health care," and so will not be paid for.
- *Shift Costs to Employees.* In order to make users of care more sensitive to costs and less profligate in their demands for care, make them pay more — either by increasing their share of insurance premiums or by increasing "copayment" out of pocket at the point of service.

So far, these efforts to limit health care costs, at least insofar as they have really been tried, have largely failed. The inflation of the health care bill remains a fact of life, and a second round of cost-cutting maneuvers, likely more painful than the first, seems inevitable.

The failure of cost containment is, in fact, a double failure. Not only has the hemorrhage of dollars continued, but the new financial ground rules have created new worries about the quality of the system. The same payers who have urged that doctors and hospitals bear greater financial risk so that they will be more sensitive to costs now worry that those providers of care will cut quality corners as they try to save dollars. The fear is aggravated by the lack of conventions and methods for assessing health care quality. Prepayment, cost shifting, competition, and the like — tools for making providers and patients more sensitive to cost — are all shooting in the dark when it comes to quality; no one yet knows their real, long-run effects on the quality of care. Payers have become afraid of the darkness.

However painful it was financially to support physicians who could get paid for anything they wished to do, it is worrisome in quite a different way to wonder if the doctors in a prepaid system might withhold needed care because they stand to gain financially from doing so. Suddenly, the link between cost control and quality seems stark. Will quality survive?

Variation in Clinical Practice

Other forces have helped push quality to the forefront of concern as well. By the late 1970s, a maturing line of investigation in health services research was bearing a message no one was happy to hear — namely, that almost anywhere one looks in health care, variability in patterns of clinical practice is rampant. That message, brought first by Dartmouth Medical School's intrepid John Wennberg, would have been laughed at two decades earlier, but Wennberg's evidence has been overwhelming.

The variation exists equally at any level of magnification of the system under study. It has been found in comparisons of Norway to New England, California to Massachusetts, one county in Vermont to another, one hospital in Boston to its neighbor, one doctor to another within a group practice, and even in the practice of a single doctor from one patient to the next. This is not subtle, marginal variation, either; it is slam-dunk variation — commonly twofold and threefold differences in rates of test ordering, surgery, drug use, and hospitalization. Wennberg found that, in one county in Maine, 70 percent of women had had hysterectomies by the age of seventy; in a nearby county, the figure was only 20 percent.

The measured variation has survived all efforts of statistical housekeeping to adjust for possible explanatory facts about the patients: age, diagnosis, socioeconomic status, level of severity. If Wennberg is right—and others have followed with similar findings—then the health care dollar is not only inflating, it is being spent largely in some colossal game of dice. The care patients receive apparently depends in large measure on who happens to be treating them. The evidence on variation makes simple trust in the quality of care seem naive.

Medicine for Profit

The arrival in force of "for-profit" medicine has also increased concern about quality. A fraction of hospitals have been run for profit for many decades, but under the new regulatory rules of the 1980s—designed to encourage competition in order to hold down prices—investor-owned health care organizations have found new life. Enormous hospital chains have formed, paying dividends to stockholders and subject to the pressures of Wall Street. Major national health maintenance organizations are similarly organized.

This corporatization of health care in for-profit companies accompanies parallel changes in the voluntary sector, as not-for-profit health care organizations have realized that their survival depends on professional management and that physicians are not necessarily the best managers. By 1985, 46 percent of physicians leaving training became employees of some health care organization, not self-employed professional entrepreneurs. Arrowsmith's shingle is becoming an antique; solo private practice, a thing of the past.

Practicing on their own, doctors who collect their patients' payments are, of course, "for profit," too. The doctor's income is profit. But, heretofore, something in the mystique of medicine, perhaps in the handshake between doctor and patient, preserved a fact or an illusion: that the doctor was motivated by the patient's interests, income notwithstanding.

In fact, considerable evidence points to the power of the profit motive even in solo medical practice. Medical procedures, for example, are often widely used and charged for long before their clinical utility is proved. Outmoded practices, whose worth has long since been disproved by scientific evidence, tend to remain in use for many years. Nonetheless, in the main, patients have trusted physicians to do their best, not to earn their most.

But can patients trust "the company" equally? Can they trust the doctor *as employee?* New structures might imply new loyalties. For example, does the physician drawing a salary, including a bonus plan that depends on the year-end bottom line, still regard the patient as the only client? Do the managers newly in charge, with M.B.A.'s and not M.D.'s after their names, really understand health care well enough to make safe and wise choices about patient care? Do stockholders want the hospitals they own to defend care at all costs, or do they expect first to see a sound quarterly dividend? If loyalties are thus realigned, is it safe to leave the physicians and hospitals in charge as the sole, and implicit, arbiters of quality?

Malpractice

In 1980, three out of every 100 American physicians were sued by patients. In 1985, eleven out of every 100 were sued. In 1989, the annual malpractice premium of a Long Island obstetrician, neurosurgeon, or orthopedist commonly exceeded $150,000. The trend toward liability litigation is noticeable in other sectors of American enterprise, as well, but in health care it marks a new level of suspicion and distance between doctors and patients.

Regulation

Suspicion is reflected, too, in the climate of health care regulation. Almost every level of government is moving more deeply into surveillance of both care and finance in medicine. For example, the Health Care Financing Administration (HCFA) — the federal agency that buys health care for the elderly under Medicare and for others under various versions of federal health insurance — maintains an elaborate network of contracts for the

review of hospital and HMO care received by Medicare bene-
ficiaries. In an effort to provide "better information for consumers," HCFA has also used its enormous database of claims
information to publish annually case-mix adjusted mortality rates
for each of nearly 6,000 American hospitals for several categories
of diseases among elderly people admitted to each hospital. By
1987, thanks to HCFA, the morning paper could publish the
rank of the local hospital, among all American hospitals, in death
rates for the care of coronary artery disease, for example. HCFA
has cautioned that the death rates should not necessarily be used
to draw conclusions about quality. Some find that caution dis-
ingenuous or at least ineffective, and the hospitals are frightened. The discussion, like it or not, *is* about quality.

In New York State, the Commissioner of Public Health
has issued a series of regulations of unprecedented scope requiring hospitals to report untoward incidents to the state. In Massachusetts, the Board of Registration in Medicine, which licenses
physicians to practice, has required that each hospital and clinic
notify the Board when any employed physician is placed under
scrutiny for possible errors in care. In these states, and in a growing number of others, governmental agencies are reaching into
the implicit quality control measures claimed by the profession.
Implicit is no longer good enough; quality is now an explicit
issue. The Physicians' Lounge is under surveillance.

Wanted: A Way to Measure Quality

As the floodlights turn on, and in the ensuing fear, medicine and its clients have become aware that *neither* has the tools
to accomplish the explicit assessment of quality of care. In the
hands of the profession as the dominant authority, health care
did not seem to need explicit quality measurement. The profession did its own surveillance, or claimed to, using back room
processes — collegial processes. The brotherhood washed its own
linens; when a brother wandered, he was corrected or removed
with the privacy and dignity befitting a trusted profession. Surveillance happened from within, and that was enough.

With the new accountability — to payers, regulators, and
lawyers, for example — the professional rites of surveillance no

longer suffice. Managers, regulators, payers, and patients demand data on quality, lest they be unable to seek and defend what they value. Professionals, reactively, have developed an interest in such data, too, lest they be unable to defend what *they* value.

But the tools are missing. They have never been built. "Quality assurance" in health care, though it is a topic with a considerable academic pedigree, never became an applied technology under the old ground rules. The research literature on quality assurance is abundant but generally unsuitable for day-to-day use. It tends toward arcane language, slow methods, and high levels of aggregation; it speaks more to scientists than to managers.

Elegant in its own way as a descriptive science, academic quality assurance has one other serious flaw: *It lacks a general theory of the sources of hazard in the complex processes of care.* On the whole, to the extent that quality measurement tools have been developed at all, they tend to unveil the *fact* of flaw, not its *cause.*

Avedis Donabedian, the founder of the field of health care quality assurance as a recognizable discipline, offered the categories of "structure," "process," and "outcome" as the three potential targets of the assessment of care. *Structures* are the resources assembled to deliver care, such as the credentials of doctors, the characteristics of buildings, and the standard procedures as specified. *Process,* in Donabedian's lexicon, means "the care itself"—which medicines are used, how diagnoses are made, which procedures are performed. *Outcomes* are the valued results of care, such as lengthening life, relieving pain, or satisfying the consumer of care.

Hundreds of research papers have been written trying to define sound structures, good processes, and suitable outcomes, along with approaches to their measurement. Hundreds more have sought links among the three, usually guided by the notion that outcomes are the "ideal" targets of measurement, and that structures and processes are interesting only to the extent that they are known to be connected to certain outcomes.

Inside health care organizations, "quality assurance" has generally been another matter entirely, bearing little connection to the academic field. The Quality Assurance Committee,

meeting in a community hospital to review the untimely death
of a twenty-three-year-old anthropology student with cancer,
probably pays little attention to the work of Donabedian, or of
any of the other deacons of the field from which the committee
took its name. They work as a good club works — serious, car-
ing, social, bound to their own local tradition and using their
own local methods. Donabedian has little to do with them. And
neither Donabedian nor the Quality Assurance Committee seems
adequate at all to the payers and regulators of health care, with
their pressing needs in the worrisome 1990s.

New Rules, Old Assumptions

None of the three — the academic researchers, the traditional quality assurance review processes, or the querulous out-
siders — has what they really need to cope with the 1990s: They
have neither tools nor theory. They *do* have assumptions about
quality and its defense, but the assumptions lack the discipline
of managerial expertise and the backbone of axiomatic logic.
The assumptions are rooted in the past, a past in which the doctor ruled. Strangely, those assumptions have survived the revo-
lutions that now deny the doctor the sole authority to judge and
guide care.

The doctor no longer really controls health care, as in the
days of solo practice, but, when it comes to quality, the doctor
is still held accountable. When the researchers study quality,
they focus on the behavior of the physician. When the Quality
Assurance Committee meets, it reviews the performance of the
physician. When the payers and the regulators turn on their
searchlights, they want doctors in their glare. Control is shifting, structure is shifting, the pattern of care is shifting; but accountability is not.

Quality Management in Industry

While American health care is engaged in its late-twen-
tieth-century revolution, a different revolution (but one also
closely linked to cost) is underway in other industries. Those

industries have had outside catalysts, most significantly the Japanese.

In 1950, "made in Japan" meant "junk," and if you could make something in America, you could sell it. Chevrolets were backordered many months; you waited for your new car and you were happy just to get it.

By 1989, things were different. Honda was on its way to becoming the third largest automobile manufacturer in America; eight out of the top ten cars as rated by American drivers were Japanese or German. Entire product lines—videocassette recorders, single lens reflex cameras, compact disc players— did not have a single American manufacturer. The top three recorders of American patents in 1989 were Japanese companies. The balance of trade threatens the life-style of America, and American capital assets are being sold at an alarming rate to finance our inefficiency.

As it has risen to prominence in health care, quality has also risen to the top of the agenda of American industry. In health care, the quality crisis is one of lost trust and shaken confidence; in manufacturing and non–health care service industries, it is a matter of survival.

Unlike health care, however, as American manufacturing companies became aware that quality and survival are linked, they did not enter a vacuum of theory and technique. To be sure, the American "Quality Control Department," much like the hospital "Quality Assurance Committee," had been operating in old and habitual modes that seemed unequal to the challenges ahead. But the *field* had not stagnated as an applied science.

On the contrary, the field of industrial quality control had flowered with new theory and technique through the entire period of decay of the dominant position of American industry. Ironically, that flowering had begun largely in the United States; we incubated the seeds of our own undoing. For, while American industry was complacent in the 1950s and 1960s, it was nurturing in a few of its back rooms the very same engineers and theoreticians of quality who, finding no pulpit in this country, were sent at government expense (*our* government) in the

early 1950s to Japan to assist in the reconstruction of its battered economy. Between 1950 and 1975, Americans learned little
from these quality pioneers, while Japan listened carefully to
what they taught.

What they taught was that quality improvement guided
by theory and systematic information can help complex systems
of production to function at levels of quality, efficiency, productivity, and morale that usually cannot even be imagined in systems "improved" by misguided intuition and habitual forms of
control. They believed that the systematic improvement of quality can be not simply an art, but a managerial science guided
by theories grounded in statistics, engineering, psychology, and,
most of all, hard-won experience.

They taught that experimentation can help production
if it is demystified and brought outside the laboratory and onto
the shop floor. They demonstrated that the greatest asset of any
production system is the human thinkers in it, and that these
thinkers are everywhere, ready, with proper leadership, to con-
vey their ideas into action. In the view of these experts the
challenge of managing quality is not one of control, but one of
enabling; quality defects generally come not from workers, but
from the systems into which those workers are placed by managers; and blame, discipline, and exhortation have little to offer
in the pursuit of better quality.

They discovered that actions of managers to improve quality without proper theory can easily cause quality to decay, not
improve, as fear and waste result. Actions uninformed by theory they called "tampering," and tampering does not build, it
destroys.

They showed the deep theoretical link between quality,
on the one hand, and process variation, on the other. Unpredictable processes do not lead to consistently excellent quality. Controlling quality means, in part, managing processes so that they
become predictable.

These new experts suggested that the proper quest for
quality is not a matter of thresholds, standards, inspection, and
certification — not a series of decisions to accept or reject a tele-
vision set, or an employee, or, for that matter, a doctor — but

rather a continuous search for small opportunities to reduce waste, rework, and unnecessary complexity. The pursuit of quality in their hands became incremental, not dramatic.

American industry remained relatively unaware of the achievements of quality control theory and application while the Japanese were working their revolution; American health care remained totally oblivious to it. That is not surprising, since the language of quality control, as developed by Walter Shewhart at Bell Telephone Laboratories and those who followed him — like W. Edwards Deming, Joseph Juran, Kaoru Ishikawa, and George Box — did not invite analogy to medicine. These experts wrote about "processes" in production (a use of the word very different from Donabedian's "processes" of care), "statistical control," "defects," "customers," "suppliers," and "costs of poor quality." Who in medicine would find it obvious that an internist's referral to an orthopedist is accomplished through a "production process," that "defects" are as inevitable in health care as they are in any complex system, that patients are usually "customers" and that nurses often are, or that surgeons and laboratories are "suppliers" bound in interdependence? What medical organization would easily discover that the "costs of poor quality" in health care are everywhere high, or believe that, as the quality of care rises, the costs of care will truly fall?

Health care organizations, in sum, have not come to believe that improving quality is, for them, necessary for survival.

Moreover, a central tenet of quality improvement theory, that quality is made not by people but by processes, flies in the face of a central myth of health care — that quality is made by doctors. Any medical leader who had discovered Deming's work in 1960 (and no one appears to have done so) would have found it irrelevant, since that leader would have been quite sure that health care depended, first and last, on physicians' doing their work properly. The buck stopped with the doctor, period. Doctors were trained to believe themselves completely responsible for the care they gave, and patients wanted that to be so. Seeing health care as a "production process" by any name would have violated both the self-image of the profession and the desires of the patients.

It is midnight and the new intern is meeting with the supervising junior resident. The intern has just done a spinal tap on a patient with suspected meningitis.

"What did the spinal fluid show under the microscope?" the junior resident asks.

"I'm not sure yet," the intern answers. "The laboratory hasn't phoned down its report."

"That answer is completely unacceptable," the junior resident chides. "That is *your* patient in there, and so far as you can be concerned, nobody has looked at the spinal until you, yourself, have. Do it. Now, Doctor."

The junior resident did not phrase it this way, but might have: "Never, Doctor, accept a role as a component of a system producing care. Your identity as a physician should always reflect the theory that you, and you alone, are responsible for the care of the patient. You are a cog in nothing, a piece of nothing. The care stems from you; you take the burden, you take the credit, and, if it fails, you take the blame." It is a wonderful message. It is full of drama, motivation, pride, control, authority, and generosity.

It is also wrong. Walk the halls of the modern hospital, past imaging machines, specialized wards, scurrying doctors, and glowing monitors. Open a patient's chart, containing hundreds of test reports, a dozen consultation notes, computerized pharmacy sheets, page after page of writing and thinking. See the patient, the victim of one among thousands of possible illnesses, in complicated stages, with multiple comorbidities. Follow the pathways of care among specialists, among hospitals, between outpatient and inpatient facilities. Notice the technologies, the people, the departments, the pace. In the hospital of the 1990s, can any one person be held totally accountable for the care we create together? Or is that the ideal of a romantic past, which no longer serves patients well in the complex present?

The night custodian bends down and throws out the trash—an errant unused X-ray report. Before it was trash, it could have saved a life. Will it happen again? How will we stop it?

We need knowledge. We need instruments for adaptation and change. We need theory. What we do is too important to let our pride keep us from lessons that have been taught and learned outside medicine about how quality can be planned, controlled, and improved. This book is intended to open some doors to those lessons, and to test their applicability to a health care system for which old ways of reacting may not be good enough anymore.

2

Applying Quality Management to Health Care

A physician manager returned recently from a visit to an American manufacturing company famous for its investment in modern quality management methods.

"I went into a back office area to look around," he said, "and the first thing I noticed was the walls. They didn't just have pictures on them; they were full of hand-drawn graphs and charts. I interrupted a clerk and asked her what the charts were all about. She said they were her 'control charts,' and that she used them to make sure that her office systems were functioning properly.

"I asked her when her training in quality improvement started. 'The day I arrived,' she told me, 'but it has really never stopped since.'"

Visit any such company, and there are lots of surprises in store. The employees at all levels, like the clerk just mentioned, seem to value data about their own work. They seek such data; they collect them as part of their jobs; they interpret them; and they use them daily. For them, "management reports" are a service, not a surveillance system.

This active use of information is only the beginning of what is new. Ask the employees about the purpose of their company, and you may be surprised to discover that they have detailed knowledge of it. You will find a consistency of vision up and down the hierarchical ladder; people know their jobs and know why their jobs exist. They are also aware of their interdependencies. Employees in manufacturing areas understand the work of support services; the business office understands the front line; the design people understand production, and production people speak regularly with designers. You will have a hard time finding people who blame each other for their troubles at work.

Ask the employees who their customers are, and they will tell you clearly. Ask them what the customers need, and they will tell you that, too, since they have asked the same questions themselves and actively sought the answers.

Ask workers chosen at random when they last served on a quality improvement team, and they are likely to say they are on one now. In the team, they meet regularly with people from other departments and other organizational levels in order to accomplish a specific, time-limited goal for which the team was created by a management council: to improve a particular process on which quality depends. The team members have received specific training in quality improvement methods; they have learned how to define problems, create hypotheses, collect data, analyze the data, and design and test remedies. They are making their own work, and the work of others, better.

Ask them how the company can afford to give them the time to serve on teams, and they will ask how the company could afford *not* to.

Not surprisingly, morale is high. The company can report steadily decreasing employee turnover ever since it got serious about quality improvement, and the unions, instead of obstructing change, are helping to lead the effort. The employees are sharing financially in the growing profits of the company; but, as you study their faces, you will begin to wonder if it really *is* profit and income that these workers are enjoying so much.

No organization is perfect, but the combination of statistical thinking, customer orientation, teamwork, clarity of mission, pride, continuous improvement, and profitability that the preceding image suggests is found increasingly often among modern companies that have learned how to manage and improve the quality of products and services. In astonishing measure, this is how the quality leaders of today—Sony, Mitsubishi, Honda, Toyota, Florida Power and Light, Bridgestone Tire, Motorola, Xerox, and many others—*really* function. This need not be taken on faith; you can visit these companies and see for yourself.

Now imagine a hospital that runs this way. Imagine its X-ray department, for example. On the walls of the X-ray department offices are numerous charts and graphs. One, labeled "Receipt of Reports by Primary Care Physicians," is maintained by the clerical supervisor, who samples performance twice each week with the help of the supervisor in the internal medicine department. It is a "control chart," showing the number of X-ray reports that fail to reach the ordering physician. The chart has been kept for almost two years, and for most weeks during that time the number of failed receipts (out of each sample of 100) is "0" or "1." Occasionally it is "2," "3," or "4," and very rarely, "5." One week stands out from earlier in the year: "10" reports lost.

"We tracked that down right away," announces the night supervisor proudly. "It was clearly a special cause. Turned out that a new mailroom clerk thought that all X-ray reports went to medical records first; we had forgotten to tell him the correct path. The poor guy felt awful, but we told him it wasn't his fault at all. Blaming never gets us anywhere."

The control system for report receipt was developed from the work of a quality improvement team three years earlier. There had been no specific problem about X-ray reporting, but a joint meeting of the radiology and internal medicine departments had used the nominal group method to identify high-priority processes for improvement. (Such joint meetings occur frequently among many departments in this hospital; that is how they best come to understand each other's needs.) The reporting process was one of the key ones identified, and the health center management committee had immediately charged a team to study and improve it. On the team were the chief of radiology, an internist, a pediatrician, a radiology technician, two ward clerks, a supervisor from the mailroom, a medical records librarian, and the assistant director of the computer services department. (At any particular time, the hospital — which has about 1,200 employees — has about 60 such teams in action. Every employee, including the hospital's executives, serves on at least one team every two years.)

The Radiology Reporting team had met weekly for four months before it held its final celebration, and it suggested six improvements in the reporting process, none of which required more staff or space. The health center management committee helped the team implement all six recommendations. The team documented that improving the process reduced lost reports from an average of 7 per 100 to slightly less than 1 per 100. (No one could figure out why there had not been more complaints when 7 out of 100 were being lost, except that lost reports had, by then, become a familiar part of work.)

Now, three years later, the control charts show that the new level of performance is still being achieved, although recently there has been discussion of appointing a new team to try to reduce lost reports by tenfold, to an average of 1 in 1,000. The process owner (the radiology supervisor) likes the idea, which was originally suggested by a secretary in internal medicine, and has nominated it to the quality council.

In a nearby town, a recent graduate of an anthropology doctoral program, whose education had been briefly interrupted by curative treatment for stage II lymphoma — which was discovered on a routine chest X-ray — is nursing her three-month-old baby.

In the hospital, in the on-call room of the intensive care unit, a senior resident is sleeping soundly. There is no cardiac arrest, and no helpless watching as a missed diagnosis works its way toward disaster. The Quality Assurance Committee has no death to review, and no one to blame or exculpate. The senior resident and the anthropology student have never even met.

This is a hospital that prevents its own failures. It heals itself. It knows how to.

Will It Work in Health Care?

It is natural to wonder if the methods of industrial quality management really can help in health care. The differences seem profound between the modern hospital and the modern factory, even more so between the assembly line and the doctor's office.

The question is important; the stakes are high. In manufacturing, quality management has yielded impressive dividends in product performance, customer satisfaction, and company profitability. In five years, Motorola used quality management to move from the brink of bankruptcy to worldwide market dominance, and, in 1988, won the first-ever National Quality Award from the U.S. Department of Commerce. Ford Motor Company used quality management methods to move from losses of $3.6 billion in 36 months between 1980 and 1982 to the highest automobile company profits ever seen in this country. Quality management methods took Bridgestone Tire Company from near shambles to the fastest growth rate in its industry. The excellence of Japanese electronic products like videocassettte recorders and 35-mm cameras has practically driven American companies from the field of competition.

What if this were possible in health care, too? Could hospitals, managed with quality improvement methods, also achieve new levels of efficiency, patient satisfaction, safety, clinical effectiveness — and profitability? Could the health care industry, battered by reactions to its rising costs and its variable performance, find in quality improvement methods at least one promising answer to its persistent problems?

The reasons for skepticism are many:

- Doesn't quality management apply only when there is a standard, uniform product? How can it help in medical care where every patient is different?
- Where is the assembly line in health care? Isn't quality mainly a matter of the doctor's making the correct decision?
- Quality management certainly helped under the cultural rules in Japan, but how can it work in the individualistic culture of the United States?
- Doctors do not like to see themselves as team players in organizations. How can quality management work with physicians?

- Quality management requires that quality be measured. How can we possibly measure or even define something as subtle as "quality" in health care?
- Isn't the real problem not quality, but cost? The trouble is that doctors and patients want to use every technology available, while the public and industry are unwilling to pay for it. Won't higher quality mean higher costs?

The National Demonstration Project:
An Experiment in the Application of
Quality Management to Health Care

Over 100 clinicians, health care executives, and industrial quality control professionals had many of these questions in mind—reflecting both skepticism and hope—when they assembled in Boston in September 1987 for the inaugural meeting of the National Demonstration Project (NDP) on Quality Improvement in Health Care. They were there to begin an experimental trial of the applicability of quality management methods in some real health care organizations.

Specifically, the NDP brought together twenty-one experts in quality management from major American companies, universities, and consulting firms, and matched them with leadership teams representing twenty-one American health care organizations—hospitals, health maintenance organizations, and group practices. The quality experts were being asked to offer their expertise and tools to a health care firm willing to try them. The health care participants' assignment was to arrive in Boston with a brief statement of an internal quality problem in their organization that had to date eluded solution.

At the September 1987 planning conference, twenty-one "arranged marriages" occurred. Each industrial expert was introduced to a team from one health care organization, and together they set to work to try out quality management methods in the health care setting. In two days of workshops and training sessions at the initial conference each team produced a formal statement of the issue to be tackled, a work plan, and an agreement to return to Boston eight months later to report on progress at a summative conference. Costs were underwritten by The John A. Hartford Foundation, a leading supporter of health services research in the United States, but the time of all experts and organizational leaders was donated.

Analyzing the experiences of these pioneering project teams, based on their own written and oral reports submitted in June 1988, this book attempts to answer the question: Can modern quality management methods help in health care, and, if so, how? In the chapters that follow, we use information from the project teams' reports to inform broader discussions of the history and core concepts of modern quality management. We quote directly and often from many of those reports, illustrating many points in the teams' own words whenever possible. We try to draw lessons from the actual project team experiences. (Not all of the twenty-one original NDP teams actually completed and reported on an improvement project. Some focused on strategic planning and other issues in quality not directly pertinent to this book, and two had to abandon participation in NDP due to unanticipated internal changes. In actual fact, the examples used in this book are drawn from seventeen of the original twenty-one teams, though *all* of the participants contributed, through their experiences, to the lessons learned in this project.)

What the Demonstration Project Did Not Do

In an eight-month demonstration project much was possible, but some things were not. Two gaps, in particular, deserve mention here, lest the reader be disappointed later on.

First, although quality management *in principle* can be used to improve clinical processes, such as physician decision making, diagnostic strategies, and medical treatments, only a few project teams actually ventured into clinical terrain. For example, one team tried to improve the consistency of use of ultrasounds in pregnancy; another, the transport of critically ill infants; and a third, the use of portable X-rays. However, most of the teams stayed on the comfortable fringes, working on problems in medical organizations that more directly resembled quality problems in other industries. One studied Medicare billing; another worked on appointment waiting times; three joined forces to look at patient discharge processes; and one addressed the hiring and retaining of nurses.

That these latter teams in general succeeded reflects their hard work, but in one sense their success is no surprise at all. The evidence that quality management can help in manufacturing and business processes is overwhelming, and it is a very safe bet that the analogous processes in health care (billing, information transfer, equipment maintenance, and the like) stand to gain just as much. How different can a hospital billing office be from the billing department of any large manufacturer or retailer? The same goes for *service* processes, like making appointments, providing telephone access, and moving patients efficiently from place to place. If Four Seasons Hotels can use quality management methods to improve room turnover, or American Express to improve telephone response time, or Federal Express to improve shipping, then the patient turnover, access, and delivery processes of hospitals and health maintenance organizations are also plausible targets.

It requires a little more imagination to see how quality management can help technical medical care, and the initial work of the NDP project teams frankly falls short of proving the point. The success of the NDP projects suggests that, *even if* business and service processes were the *only* loci in health care where quality management helps, the methods would still be worth adopting in health care organizations. However, the potential for quality management extends far beyond that. The safety of patients *must* depend on the reliability of the systems that deliver their care. The appropriateness and efficiency of the decisions doctors reach *must* depend on the fidelity of the systems that deliver information, training, supplies, and options to doctors. It *must* be true that technical care that is prompt, appropriate, effective, and respectful of patients can best occur in medical organizations whose processes are streamlined, carefully designed, continuously improved, and responsive to the needs of both patients and health care workers. Yet these areas still await complete exploration.

Not a single NDP team measured its success in terms of improved health status of patients. That somewhat disappointing fact is a product, in part, of the short time frame of the demonstration project, and of the neophyte qualifications (and a certain cautiousness) of the health care teams. Future projects, in more mature quality management cultures, will discover that quality improvement helps clinical care itself.

The NDP had a second limitation: It could not try to change organizational cultures. The tools of quality improvement are very powerful, but, while they thrive in some organizational cultures, they wither in others. In its fullest form, quality management involves the "transformation" of organizations through the adoption of management methods that allow quality improvement activities to flourish. "Transformation" involves, for example, increasing the opportunities for people from different departments and functions to meet and work directly with each other, clarifying the organization's mission and translating it so that every employee can see how his or her job fits in, increasing the priority given to training and education of all employees, especially in applied statistical methods, and abolishing numerical goals and production quotas in favor of a more comprehensive emphasis on improving quality.

For most organizations, this cultural change is difficult, and the effort produces resistance. Most experts say that it takes several years for the "new" quality culture to take root. The NDP participants had only eight months in which to do their work; this is not enough time to change the culture of an organization. This report on their experiences therefore deals mainly not with fundamental organizational change, but with the use of technical methods to solve specific problems.

How This Book Is Organized

Using the work of NDP teams as examples, this book offers a picture of the basic, early steps in applying quality improvement methods in medical organizations.

Chapter Three, "Foundations of Quality Management," reviews the history and presents the theoretical model of quality management as it has developed outside health care over five decades. It introduces the basic terminology of quality management, which is necessary because this terminology encodes the new ways of thinking that guide the improvement effort.

Chapters Four through Eight present five basic steps in the technical approach to process improvement as used in virtually all organizations that manage quality in the modern mode. These chapters draw on the specific experiences of the NDP teams as they worked their way through those steps:

- Chapter Four, "Using the Scientific Method to Define Problems," shows how the team or individual develops a clear, specific statement of the goals of the improvement project
- Chapter Five, "Organizing Quality Improvement Teams," discusses cross-functional teams, how they are organized, and how they do their work
- Chapter Six, "The Diagnostic Journey," covers the methods through which teams assess symptoms, document processes, and develop and test hypotheses about the root causes of quality problems
- Chapter Seven, "Implementing Successful Remedies," demonstrates how improvements in processes are planned, implemented, and tested
- Chapter Eight, "Holding and Extending the Gains," emphasizes the preservation of improvements once they are shown to work

The model of improvement through which we discuss the work of the NDP teams is not that of any particular school or leader in the quality movement. It is quite general, sharing common ground with the ideas of W. Edwards Deming, Joseph M. Juran, Kaoru Ishikawa, George Box, and many others among the leading theoreticians and teachers in quality management. That so many different quality experts in the NDP drew from a common pool of technique to assist their health care partners attests to the ecumenical core of theory that underlies modern quality management. All schools of thought share one basic approach: scientific thinking at all levels of the organization in the continuous improvement of the processes through which work is done.

- Chapter Nine, "Ten Key Lessons for Quality Improvement," reviews the overall experience of the NDP to extract lessons for future quality management efforts in health care. What works well? What does not? What modifications will be needed in theory and technique in order for health care to take full advantage of the sciences of quality planning, improvement, and control? Most of all, what benefits can we expect? Is modern quality management only a fad — at best only a dram of relief for a threatened industry — or does it promise more substantial gains that can help health care as deeply and as durably as it has helped other industries to survive other threats?

The afterword offers some reflective comments by one quality management expert, David Garvin of the Harvard Business School, who observed and helped guide the National Demonstration Project as a member of its advisory committee.

Resource A at the back of the book lists all of the participants in the NDP, whose enthusiastic volunteer activities made this story possible.

Resource B is a comprehensive discussion of the statistical tools commonly used in early stages of quality improvement. This review of tools, more systematic and detailed than in the earlier discussions of the NDP projects, is the work of our colleague Paul E. Plsek, a consultant in quality management and a team member in one of the NDP projects.

Resource C contains three complete project team reports from the NDP, selected as representative of the work of the most successful teams. These stories, told in the teams' own words, give more texture and context to the excerpts used in the remainder of the book and present images of the entire problem-solving effort of a team from beginning to end.

Resource D provides some suggestions for further reading.

3

Foundations of
Quality Management

Quality Management: Rx for U.S. Industry

During the 1980s, in the face of fierce competition, many industrial companies in the United States adopted systematic programs of quality management. They applied quality management not just in their manufacturing operations, but in every business process in the company: marketing, finance, patent offices, sales and service, shipping, research and development labs, and white-collar administrative offices. For some of these companies, changing the ways they managed quality was not just a matter of increasing market share or decreasing costs; it was a matter of survival.

The successes achieved by many companies as a result of quality management have been spectacular. The Xerox Corporation has regained market share from its worldwide competitors. In small copiers—a market that analysts had ceded to Xerox's aggressive Japanese competitors—Xerox doubled its market share from 1979 to 1986. In one of the toughest businesses in the world, manufacturing nuclear fuel, the Westinghouse Commercial Nuclear Fuel Division has taken over 40 percent of the U.S. market and over 20 percent of the world market. After achieving a ten-to-one improvement in the reliability of nuclear fuel cells (from 99.95 to 99.995 percent) in just three years, Westinghouse has set a new goal of another ten-to-one improvement in the next year alone. In electronics, probably the American industry whose precarious situation has received the most publicity, Motorola is not only generating record profits, but is today the world leader in cellular telephones and is rapidly approaching its explicit corporate goal of quality defect levels of approximately three parts per million — performance unimaginable only a few years ago.

What do these companies have in common? First, they are among the initial winners of the Malcolm Baldrige National Quality Award. Second, they are all engaged in comprehensive programs of strategic quality management. These companies all began with modest quality improvement programs, then extended those programs to all locations and all functions. In so doing, they have provided an excellent road map for other companies — including health care organizations — to follow.

A Brief History of Quality Management

The modern approach to quality management is the product of a long evolution. For centuries, the only form of "quality management" was inspection. Early craftspeople inspected their own work or that of apprentices they directly observed. As shops grew in size, and as production became standardized in the era of the management scientist Frederick Taylor and the industrialist Henry Ford, direct supervision by craftspeople was no longer practical; a separate inspection function was created. Inspectors were trained to study the outcomes of work, often armed with sophisticated statistical methods for deciding just how many samples to inspect from a lot and when to pass or discard the entire lot based on results from the sample. Inspection added costs, but it was considered necessary in order to protect customers from defective products.

By the mid 1920s, inspection itself came under scrutiny, most significantly in Walter Shewhart's path-breaking book, *The Economic Control of the Quality of Manufactured Product* (1931). In a major change in philosophy, Shewhart's work suggested that the efforts of a company be directed not at finding and fixing problems in the *products,* but rather at finding and fixing problems in the *processes* of work. Proper control of the processes of production, he argued, was far more efficient than endpoint inspection in assuring and improving quality.

Quality control methods in accordance with Shewhart's theory developed quickly in Great Britain and the United States during World War II, but in the postwar era it was the Japanese who deployed the techniques most fully. With the assistance of American experts like W. Edwards Deming and Joseph M. Juran, the Japanese learned to apply the methods of quality control not just to manufacturing, but also to the control and improvement of design, marketing, distribution, sales, service, and all other business functions of a company.

This extension of quality control throughout a company was given new definition and emphasis by A. V. Feigenbaum in his pioneering book, *Total Quality Control* (1983). Feigenbaum proposed total quality control as a system for integrating quality-related efforts throughout an organization so that all functions could focus together on the efficient satisfaction of the customer's needs. The Japanese further expanded this concept to include participation of the entire work force in quality management, regardless of hierarchical level. In this form, companywide total quality control involved a complete mobilization of improvement and control efforts — including all levels and all functions — in one corporate effort. In its most advanced form, total quality management today involves both *horizontal* (across functions) and *vertical* (across hierarchical levels) integration of the company's strategic focus on quality.

These methods were not entirely ignored in America. They were applied, for example, in companies that were faced with the stringent quality requirements of the space program and by others that faced particularly brutal competition. Unfortunately, however, many American companies slept through the early stages of the modern quality era. They failed to recognize the emerging competition in quality: competition based on improving customer satisfaction and reducing the costs of poor quality. Many companies collapsed, lost huge chunks of market share, or simply withdrew from global competition in many

product lines. More recently, a resurgence of interest in quality management has begun in many American industrial sectors. For some companies, as we have seen, successes have already been spectacular.

Basic Principles of Quality Management

How has quality management been instrumental in trans-
forming these companies? Modern quality management is a way
of looking at the world of production — production of almost anything. The theory supplies terms to define the components and
processes of production, insights into the nature of quality and
the causes of its failures, and methods of planning, improving,
and controlling quality. Since the basic concepts were developed first in manufacturing, they have a concrete and commercial flavor, but their application need not be restricted to industry. They are lenses through which to understand the ways
productive activity occurs and can improve in *any* organization,
large or small, producing *any* kinds of goods or services.

1. Productive Work Is Accomplished Through Processes.
Quality management sees each person in an organization as part
of one or more processes. The job of every worker is to receive
the work of others, add value to that work, and supply it to the
next person in the process. This is often called the "triple role"—
the worker as customer, processor, and supplier (see Figure 3.1).
Figure 3.1 is a linear representation of the basic elements of a
process. First, we receive various kinds of *inputs* from others (that
is, *suppliers*) that we in turn use in performing our tasks; in this
sense, we are *customers* of those who provide these inputs. Next,
as *processors,* we perform various managerial, technical, or administrative tasks ("processes") using these inputs. Finally, we
act as *suppliers* to our *customers* by delivering *products* or *services*
to them. By understanding our own needs and defining them
carefully, we help our suppliers improve the quality of their
work. In the same way, by understanding the needs of our customers and defining these carefully, we improve the quality of
our own work.

Figure 3.1. The Triple Role of the Worker.

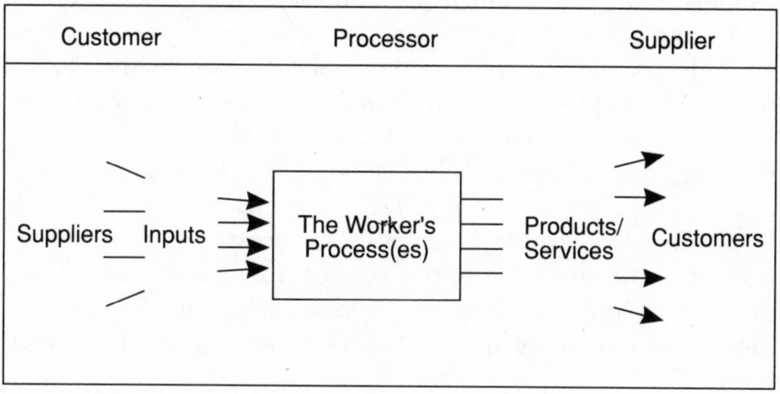

Figure 3.2 illustrates a basic production process schematically, showing how the interdependent activities within the process work together to transform inputs into outputs that customers value. Many people, working in their respective "triple roles" within the process, add value in this sequence of productive

Figure 3.2. Elements of a Process.

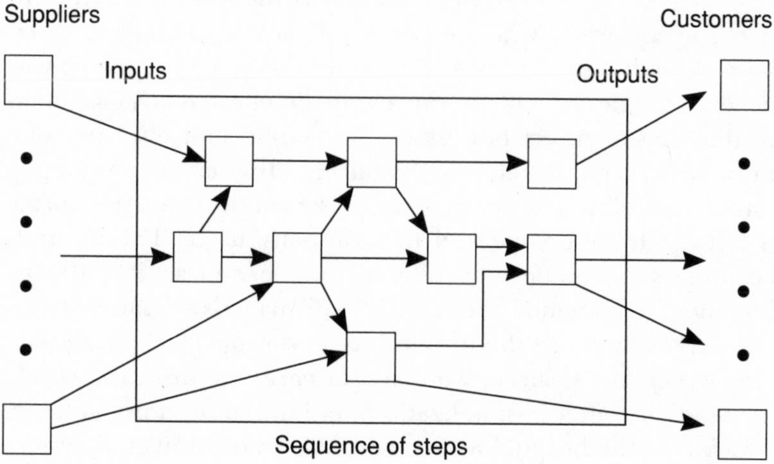

steps. Each action makes the product and service more and more valuable to the people who depend on those products and services.

Although processes are easiest to visualize in manufacturing lines, the concept is a general one, applying as well to the production of intangibles, such as information, amusement, or health. In health care, as in any complex production system, much of the work can be framed as processes, each with its own set of *customers* and *suppliers: patient flow* processes that move people from place to place, *information flow* processes that create and transport the grist for informed decisions, and *material flow* processes that move equipment and supplies. Quality management begins with seeing the world of production in process terms.

2. Sound Customer-Supplier Relationships Are Absolutely Necessary for Sound Quality Management.   Modern quality theory is "customer centered." Managing quality means trying to improve the capability and reliability of processes to meet the needs of those served by the processes. The competitive advantage for a company that can better meet the requirements of its paying customers is obvious; such a company will gain market share, can charge higher prices in accord with the higher value of its products, and can waste less effort in activities that do not add value for customers.

Less obvious are the advantages that lie in meeting the needs of customers who are not simply buyers of goods and services. Quality management defines my customer as anyone who depends on me. Manufacturing companies have many customers in this sense — direct purchasers, of course, but also the community at large, which may be affected by the company's pollution control processes, secondary users of the company's products, and the employees of the company itself. The multiple customers of a modern hospital include, of course, its patients, but they also include the families and friends of patients, the physicians who use the hospital as a workplace, the hospital's employees, the insurers who pay for care, the institutions that help patients after hospitalization, and the community at large, which sees the hospital as one component of its overall system for maintaining and restoring health.

Quality management maintains that good customer-supplier relationships — characterized by long-term commitments, clear communications, and mutual trust — are more likely to improve quality than are suspicious, transient, and anonymous relationships. This is true not only of the *external customer-supplier relationships* (those between a company and its customers) but also of so-called *internal customer-supplier relationships* (those that lie within the work process). Indeed, it is a central concept in quality management that the quality of products and services provided to the external customer is determined in large part by the quality of internal customer-supplier relationships. Modern quality management thus invests heavily in forms of interaction, measurement, and clarification of roles that can help internal customers and suppliers understand and serve each other more effectively.

Not uncommonly, a company's multiple customers have interests that are, or appear to be, in conflict. Buyers want prompt delivery, but the community wants noise abatement that requires certain hours of shut-down. Health care payers want costs controlled, but physicians want access to the most modern technologies of care. These trade-offs make quality planning difficult, but they do not change the basic premise that *the better the organization can understand and meet the needs of its diverse customers, the more successful it will be in the long run.*

3. The Main Source of Quality Defects Is Problems in the Process. When companies first analyze their critical processes, they are usually struck by how complex they are. Many processes, even some processes that are absolutely central to the success of the organization, were not designed; they just evolved. They consist of activities that grew by accretion over time and were passed on from one generation of managers and workers to the next. Once companies understand the complexities of the processes they use, with their numerous input/output sub-processes, they are not at all surprised at the frequency with which defects emerge. Indeed, they are usually more surprised that the processes work at all.

A fundamental difference between modern quality management concepts and alternative theories that emphasize the accountability of individuals for the quality of the work they do is the understanding of the importance of the system of production. Modern quality management draws on voluminous evidence that failures in quality—that is, failures to add value for customers or failures to meet customers' needs—usually can be traced to inherent flaws in the processes in which people work, not to the failure of people to do their work as they are instructed to do it. As one quality expert has put it, "The old assumption is that quality fails when people do the right thing wrong; the new assumption is that, more often, quality failures arise when people do the wrong thing right."

The correlates of this theory of flaw are several. First, the theory suggests that *exhortation, incentives, and discipline of workers are unlikely to improve quality.* If quality is failing when people do their jobs as designed, then exhorting them to "do better" is managerial nonsense. In fact, such exhortations amount to insults, since they imply, wrongly, that the defects would not arise if workers cared more.

For example, in the case in Chapter One, it is easy to blame the physician who failed to pursue the missing X-ray report on the curable cancer that later became fatal. Quality management theory suggests another approach: recognize that a flawed process is probably at work and set out to fix that process. The hypothetical physician in Chapter One is dependent on the processes through which routine X-rays are ordered, performed, and reported back. Perhaps it is a characteristic of these processes that, on average, one in a hundred routine reports never reaches the ordering doctor—or one in a thousand, or one in ten, as the case may be.

In such circumstances, no degree of exhortation or deterrence will fundamentally improve the system. Heroic thoroughness may make patients a little safer, but the important battles of improvement are not won by heroes who compensate over and over again for flawed processes. They are won by those who vanquish the real enemy: the process flaws themselves. The proper objects of efforts to improve quality are not the *people* who participate in a flawed process, but the *processes* that make flaws happen in the first place.

A second correlate is that *the responsibility for improving quality belongs to managers.* Workers in the typical company only rarely can control or change the circumstances of their own work; they usually lack the authority, security, and autonomy to do so. A solution requires managers to organize efforts to improve processes of production. Modern quality management theory has roots in the work of organizational psychologists who have claimed that substantial reservoirs of pride, competence, and aspiration exist among workers. The drive to do well is widespread. The job of leaders, then, is more to mobilize and enable the latent talents and energy of the entire work force than to ensure that people do their work properly through systems of monitoring, control, and incentive.

4. Poor Quality Is Costly.   Modern quality management seeks two types of quality improvement: improvements in quality that result from reduction in deficiencies and improvements that involve adding features that please the customer or that meet more of the customer's needs. Pursuit of the former type of quality ("freedom from deficiencies") almost always reduces costs, sometimes dramatically. Pursuit of the latter type of quality ("new features to meet customers' needs") may have advantages for an organization in gaining market share, enabling premium pricing, and increasing customer satisfaction, but it often costs more. Modern quality management involves both enterprises: finding, eliminating, and preventing deficiencies, and developing the most efficient methods to meet more customer needs.

As quality management experts came to understand that quality problems come from flaws in processes, they also developed an increasing sense of the pervasiveness of the costs of poor quality. When processes fail to meet customers' needs reliably, costs mount quickly. If the processes cannot be counted on to yield satisfactory results, companies must maintain surveillance over the results, inspecting finished products and discarding the defective ones.

Poor quality also results in a variety of internal failure costs, as the organization does what it must to repair the defects it finds. Defective products are discarded, becoming waste; new

ones must be made to replace those discarded, a form of rework; often, "Band-Aid" processes are added in an effort to inter-
cept defects, thus increasing complexity without adding real
value. Moreover, awareness of quality failure erodes pride among
workers, often decreasing their motivation or loyalty.

Quality defects almost always result in external failure
costs as well. These are costs incurred when, because no inspection is perfect, the defective product or service reaches customers.
They may become dissatisfied and tell their friends, leading to
market share losses. They may sue or ask for replacements, increasing the costs of warranty.

The intent of modern quality management is to recover
these enormous costs of inspection, external failure, and internal failure (which can easily amount to 25 or 30 percent of the
total cost of production) as much as possible by investing in the
prevention of quality failures. This requires careful attention
to the design of products and services and to the design and control of the processes through which they are made. The goal
is to prevent defects *before* they must be repaired, and to develop
and maintain processes so reliable that inspection of the end
result can be safely reduced or ultimately even eliminated.

One way to think of prevention as an approach to qual-
ity management is that *it moves inspection upstream in a process.* Inspecting end results is necessary so that the organization can
keep on its course of meeting customer needs, but relying on
endpoint inspection to achieve quality is costly and inevitably
imperfect. It is better to inspect and understand the processes
of work, so as to discover the ways in which flaws are introduced
into products and services. Better still is to have a way to inspect designs before they ever become real processes. The aim
of quality management is to "do it right the first time."

*5. Understanding the Variability of Processes Is a Key to
Improving Quality.* In every process and in every measurement, variability exists. This is well understood in many parts
of medicine. When clinical investigators conduct research trials
to determine the effectiveness of a new treatment or drug, they
design them to control as much as possible the unwanted variability contributed by differences among individuals or among

disease subgroups, for example. The researchers try to select samples large enough to reduce the effect of the sources of variation that they cannot control by design. They try to increase the "signal" and decrease the "noise" in the experiment.

In recent years, companies pursuing quality management have discovered the importance of understanding variation in the inputs and outputs of critical processes. Failure to identify and control important sources of variation is the cause of many serious quality problems. Those who manage quality learned that unpredictable processes tend to be inherently flawed. Unpredictability makes it difficult both to study and to assess the performance of a process, and to compare it with alternative processes. There is a deep relationship between experimental control of variation (for the purposes of learning) on the one hand, and managerial control of variation (for the purposes of improving quality) on the other hand. In both cases, understanding variation is a precondition to gaining knowledge about performance.

An emerging idea in quality management is the concept of *robust* quality, which suggests that it is possible to design processes to function properly even in the face of variability. For many years, companies have tried to identify the most important sources of variation and to find ways to control these sources. Although placing controls on these sources of variation has led to dramatic improvements in the quality of the final product, these controls have often proved expensive. For example, in manufacturing integrated circuits, vibration is known to cause many defects; however, reducing the many possible sources of vibration in the manufacturing plant — or isolating the chip production line — is prohibitively expensive. Designing new manufacturing processes that are less affected by the vibration is proving to be a far better solution.

6. Quality Control Should Focus on the Most Vital Processes. In quality management, it is important to identify the most important types and components of processes and control those. Those who try to control everything often find themselves buried in measurements and end up taking action on none. To assure the quality of each key parameter of a process, one must have a clear *definition* of the desired quality performance level, a way to *measure* the performance, a way to *interpret* the measurements, and a way to *take action* to reestablish control when necessary. These are the basic elements of effective quality control.

7. The Modern Approach to Quality Is Thoroughly Grounded in Scientific and Statistical Thinking. Quality management was developed by engineers, statisticians, physicists, psychologists, and others who began with a scientific question: "Why does quality fail?" These same pioneers developed the notion that the general scientific method itself held the key to improvement of processes of production.

In medicine, patients arrive with symptoms of disease; physicians engage in diagnostic efforts to find the causes; together, the doctors and patients agree on remedies to be applied and tested; and they assess the results of treatment so as to guide their next steps. In this guise, the scientific method is good medical practice.

In quality management, precisely the same method is applied. The "symptom" is a defect in quality — a failure to meet the needs of a customer. Thanks to the work of this century's quality theorists, managers can have an initial idea of the likely agent of harm: It is probably a flaw in the process of production itself. Perhaps the raw materials are defective, or the procedures are wrong, or the equipment broken, or the people improperly trained. The therapist of process, like the doctor of medicine, must perform diagnostic tests, formulate specific hypotheses of cause, test those hypotheses, design and apply remedies, and assess the effect of the remedies.

Quality management theory makes a bold suggestion; namely, it is possible and desirable for everyone in the organization to utilize the scientific method for improving processes as part of their normal daily activity. Quality management intends to place scientific tools for process improvement within the grasp of every single employee. It does this largely through extensive and regular training of all employees in quality control and improvement methods — in what George Box of the University of Wisconsin has called the "democratization of science."

This scientific approach to quality is, by its nature, based on data. Therefore, it is a characteristic of quality management to invest heavily in the design and deployment of measurement. The agenda for measurement is extensive. It must include measurement of *customer needs* ("What, exactly, do those who depend on us require?"), measurement of *inputs* ("What do we need from suppliers?" "What is being supplied?"), measurement of *process characteristics* ("Is this process stable?" "Are the activities carried out as designed?"), and measurement of *results* ("What did the customer experience?" "How did the process perform?"). Unlike other approaches to improvement, however, in which measurement is used to reward and discipline people, measurement in the quality management effort is used to gain knowledge of the processes, so that they can be understood, predicted, and improved. Measurement is used so that everyone can control and improve processes, not so that some people can control other people.

The approach to measurement in quality management is optimistic in the sense that measurement is always thought possible. Time and again, organizations have found ways to translate complex and subtle quality concepts like "reliability," "customer service," "morale," and "safety" into clear, operational measurements much as modern health services researchers have found ways to measure and represent concepts like "physical functioning," "emotional well-being," "patient satisfaction," and "activities of daily living" through carefully developed quantitative questionnaires and surveys.

8. Total Employee Involvement Is Critical.   One of the most striking discoveries of companies in the past twenty years is the power that comes from enabling all employees to become involved in quality control and improvement. It seems obvious that assuring and improving quality cannot be made the job of any single department, but for years companies (and health care organizations) tried to do just that. Organizations are now using increasingly innovative ways to encourage and capture ideas from all employees, not just from managers.

The concept of supplier-processor-customer relationships (the "triple role") and the need for numerous controls and mea-

surements throughout the organization make clear why everyone should be involved in quality control. For companies to accomplish hundreds, or even thousands, of improvement projects
a year rather than a few, they had to develop new structures
to foster employee involvement. They had to provide training
to all employees in basic methods for identifying problems or
opportunities, for discovering causes, for developing and implementing remedies, and for establishing controls at the new
levels. They also had to develop and expand the use of teams
in which employees could find opportunities to participate in
formal process improvement projects.

*9. New Organizational Structures Can Help Achieve Quality
Improvement.*   Almost all industrial companies have developed
new organizational forms to accelerate quality improvement.
First, some form of "guiding arm" or "steering committee" is advis-
able to plan the quality improvement effort strategically. Such
a "quality council" is most effective when it consists of the same
leaders who operate other key company functions. In their special
role as quality council, these leaders plan training of managers
and teams, plan the technical infrastructure for improvement,
create and maintain procedures for nomination and selection of
processes to be worked on, create and maintain forms of recognition and celebration of the work of quality improvement teams,
and evaluate and improve the quality improvement effort itself.

Most improvement occurs through special, evanescent
project teams. These teams are assembled for the purpose of
carrying out a specific improvement assignment under the authority of the quality council. The teams may be cross-functional
and may even involve members from other organizations if they
play significant roles in the processes under investigation.

These new forms — teams and councils — and the attitudes
that go with them give the quality improvement effort new vigor
and flexibility compared with formal management structures
in which most companies unaware of quality management methods are bound.

*10. Quality Management Employs Three Basic, Closely In-
terrelated Activities: Quality Planning, Quality Control, and*

Quality Improvement.   *Quality planning* involves developing a definition of quality as it applies to customers, developing measures of quality, designing products and services in accord with customer needs, designing processes capable of providing those products and services, and transferring those processes into the routine operations of the organization.

   Quality control involves developing and maintaining operational methods for assuring that processes work as they are designed to work and that target levels of performance are being achieved. Quality control requires a clear definition of quality, knowledge of expected performance or targets, measurements of actual performance, a way to compare expected to actual performance, and a way to take action when measured results are not equal to expected results, or when processes appear to be drifting from their expected performance levels.

   Quality improvement is the effort to improve the level of performance of a key process. It involves measuring the level of current performance, finding ways to improve that performance, and implementing new and better methods. Quality improvement is often where companies start first in quality management, and it is the point at which participants in the National Demonstration Project began.

The National Demonstration Project: Experiments in Quality Improvement

   The teams in the National Demonstration Project began just as Xerox, Motorola, and Westinghouse did—with basic quality improvement projects. The intent of the NDP was to help health care get started, in the belief that the best way to find out whether quality management theory and techniques were "transferable" to health care was to try them out.

   The teams followed the five basic steps—each of which corresponds to a chapter in the book—that were noted earlier:

1.   Select a problem to work on.
2.   Organize a team to carry out the improvement project.
3.   Diagnose the problem: that is, understand the process of

which it is a part and gather information on the process
in order to search for root causes of the problem.
4. Plan, test, and implement a remedy guided by process
    knowledge.
5. Check and continuously monitor performance at the new
    level, taking further action as needed to modify the remedy.

These steps in the quality improvement process are generic, and
appear in one form or another in the various models for quality improvement proposed by experts throughout industry.
Although the different labels and diagrams used by the various
consultants and teachers in this field can be confusing at first
to the newcomer, it is helpful to recognize the commonality of
the basic approaches. Figure 3.3 shows the general sequence

Figure 3.3. Steps in the QIP. (*Source:* **Juran
Institute, Inc.,** *Quality Improvement Tools,* **1989.)**

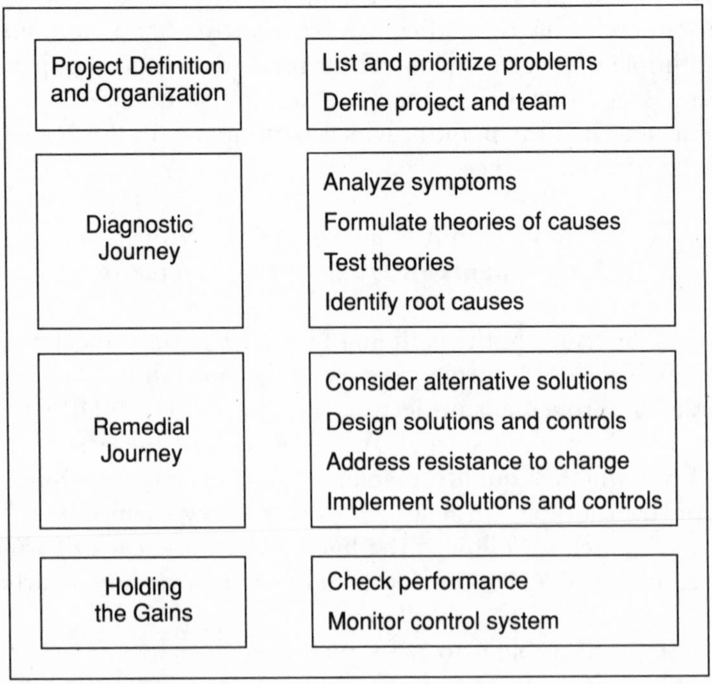

Project Definition and Organization	List and prioritize problems Define project and team
Diagnostic Journey	Analyze symptoms Formulate theories of causes Test theories Identify root causes
Remedial Journey	Consider alternative solutions Design solutions and controls Address resistance to change Implement solutions and controls
Holding the Gains	Check performance Monitor control system

of steps in the Quality Improvement Process (QIP) at a somewhat finer level of detail, and the reader can use this figure as an orienting device for the remainder of this book and, especially, for the sample project team reports in Resource C.

In Chapter Four, we begin our account of the experiences of the NDP teams as they tackled quality improvement projects, most for the first time. These experiences have the flavor of any exploration into uncharted territory: a mixture of excitement and apprehension at the start, then alternating swings of frustration and elation in the course of the journey. Above all, the teams shared a deep sense of commitment to health care and to exploring a new field full of promise to make health care better.

4   CICICICICICICICICICICICICICICI

Using the Scientific Method to Define Problems

A Clear Problem Statement: The Door to Understanding

Quality improvement uses the scientific method to understand and improve processes. Its power lies not so much in its ability to help solve any particular problem as in the *extent* of its deployment in an organization. *Everyone* in the organization — not just technical experts or high-level managers or white-collar researchers, but also hourly employees, front-line staff, people in support departments and in the business offices — *everyone* becomes, in effect, a scientist able to contribute ideas and knowledge about how work can be done more effectively. In the words of one nurse who attended an introductory course on quality management, "I get it. In this management system everyone has two jobs: their job, and the job of helping to improve their job."

The *method* of improvement is the key contribution of quality improvement: Instead of management by impulse, or by exhortation, or by preconception, the quality improvement manager is able to *manage by facts* — facts about the processes of work, and about the root causes of failures in those processes. Many organizations inside and outside health care are full of "facts" today. Reports and charts fairly spill over the edges of desks and in-baskets. But the information people really need to make what they do more effective—namely, information on *why* the processes of work are unreliable, wasteful, or otherwise frustrating to staff and customers—is missing, or is so deeply buried in the reams of other, useless numbers that real understanding of causes is nearly impossible.

In such settings, managers too often turn to exhortation. The daily report shows an apparent increase in waiting times. The manager circles the number in red pencil and sends it down the line with a note, "What happened here?" Up the line comes the answer, "Short of staff," or "Computers down," or "This number must be wrong." The real fact is that *no one knows* why waiting times have gotten longer. The information is not available to answer the question, "Why?" More important, the information is not available to guide *prevention* of trouble in the future. Ill-equipped to attack the root causes of problems, people attack the data instead, wondering if the troublesome number is merely a "fluke"; they argue that the problem is not in the process but in the measurement system.

Quality improvement as a management method seeks to organize the company in a new way—so that, in an orderly and planned fashion, *everyone at all levels can play an active role in understanding problems and the processes of work that underlie them,* collecting and analyzing data on those processes, generating and testing hypotheses about the causes of flaws, and designing, implementing, and testing remedies.

Joseph M. Juran, one of the major figures in modern quality management, suggests that improvement efforts are best conducted through specific, bounded "projects." He defines a project as "a problem scheduled for solution." W. Edwards Deming, another leader in quality management, prefers to talk about "process improvement" instead of "problem solving." Deming may want to emphasize that people should avoid dealing only with the wheels that squeak, since important opportunities for improvement may be found in processes with unrealized potential but without obvious symptoms. Whether we call the job at the start "solving problems" or "improving processes," the method is the same: act like a scientist in your daily work. State questions, make a plan, formulate hypotheses, gather data to test those hypotheses, draw conclusions, and test those conclusions.

That basic method is what the teams formed in the NDP were taught, in one way or another, by their quality advisers. This method, the *scientific method* for process improvement, begins with developing a clear statement of the problem to be worked on.

A scientist who begins her experiment without a clear statement of the question she seeks to answer will likely fail. The same is true of a quality improvement team. The first step: *Write the problem down clearly.* The initial job of the project teams was to choose and state unambiguously what they intended to work on.

Sources of Improvement Projects: Where Do the Ideas Come From?

Where do the ideas come from in the first place? And who decides which problems will be tackled first? The job of generating project ideas and choosing among them (sometimes called "nomination" and "selection") must be planned and managed in a fully developed quality improvement effort. Often, the nomination and selection process is run by a steering group of some sort — a "quality council" that sets priorities for improvement. In mature quality management efforts, this "quality council" is nothing more than the group of managers and executives who usually make other important strategic decisions for the organization. Such a steering committee may be present at many organizational levels. The corporation has its corporate quality council; a division or center has its divisional quality council; large departments have their own departmental quality councils, and so on. No matter how the organization is structured, however, *someone* — some group or individual — must design and manage the process through which ideas for improvement projects are assembled and appropriate priorities set.

Gathering Nominations by Asking the Customer

Generating enough ideas for projects is rarely a problem; but where do the best ideas come from? The answer will not surprise anyone who has studied the basic theory of quality management: The best ideas for improving organizational processes come from the *customers* who depend on the organization's products and services. The reason is simple: Quality in the modern sense is *defined* as meeting the needs of customers. Who better than the customer can tell us what is needed and how we are doing?

In health care, of course, both the idea of "customer" and the idea of "need" require some clarification. Like many other industries, health care always has multiple customers. The pediatrician serves the child, the family, the community, other physicians, nonphysician staff members, the payers (who will get the bill), and perhaps even the regulators (who need reassurance that all is well). As in other industries, health care has both *internal* and *external* customers. The former are health care workers (and processes) that depend on *other* health care workers (and processes). For example, one of the pediatrician's customers in an orthopedic referral is the consulting orthopedist; the orthopedist cannot do proper work without information supplied by the referring pediatrician. "Quality" in pediatric practice, in this regard, includes "meeting the requirements" of the (internal) customer orthopedist.

What about the *external* customer—for example, the patient with chest pain? Can we merely ask that patient how we are doing in order to find our best ideas for improvement projects? In one sense, of course, the answer is, "No," or at least, "Not exclusively." How can the patient tell us that the process of delivering oxygen therapy may be flawed, or that propranolol was administered unnecessarily or in a wrong dosage? At one level, "quality" in health care is, to the customer, opaque.

But the distinction between "perceived" and "real" (or "technical") quality becomes less distinct under a closer look. First, for a great deal of what we all would call "quality" in health care, the "customer" (patient) can both judge performance and suggest useful ideas for improvement. Most patients are perfectly capable of answering such questions as:

- "Did we answer your questions clearly?"
- "Was our service prompt enough for you?"
- "How often was your intravenous line checked during the day?"

- "Were we respectful of your privacy?"
- "How much pain did you feel?"
- "How do you feel now?"

Patients' answers to questions like these, built into standardized, formal questionnaires when possible, can provide a compass for improvement efforts in many important dimensions of quality.

Second, even for the most technical of quality issues, it is still to the patient that we must ultimately turn for evidence of quality. For example, after all of the appropriate considerations of case-mix and environmental conditions, the most important information to use in assessing the quality of anesthesia practice is the health status of the patient. The most important information to have in characterizing the results of the processes of care for heart attacks is the survival, function, and symptom level of the patients.

In the language of industrial quality management, "listening to the voice of the customer" means directly assessing the degree to which products and services are meeting the needs of those who rely on them. In health care quality, "listening to the voice of the customer" includes the systematic assessment both of the attitudes of patients and of the impact of the care processes on the health of patients. The best reporters of both attitude and health are usually patients themselves.

In medicine, the best ideas for improvement of technical care will come from listening carefully to patients about how they feel and function, and then linking their answers to the processes used in trying to change their feelings and functioning. Health care organizations that manage themselves according to quality improvement principles will inevitably develop and maintain internal systems to measure and track the health status and functioning of their patients. In the short time frame of the NDP, however, the participants could not practically develop such information systems. Nonetheless, several of the NDP teams did turn in other ways directly to customers — both internal and external ones — for guidance in choosing projects.

Listening to the External Customers

The Park Nicollet Medical Center team chose a simple method to involve external customers in defining their project. The team distributed questionnaires to over 7,000 patients, asking about their level of satisfaction with each of twenty-three different "likely causes" of dissatisfaction with ambulatory care. These "likely causes" were the result of brainstorming among team members.

When the team arrayed the responses in a simple ordered bar chart of the frequency with which each cause was mentioned by a patient (a "Pareto diagram" — see Exhibit 4.1), some surprises were in store. First, six of the twenty-three "likely" causes were cited by no patients at all. Had the team gone about to remedy those "causes" before verifying them, they would have been wasting their time. Second, as the team reported, "The ranking of 'telephone access' (that is, difficulty in getting through to a physician or having to wait too long) as the leading cause of dissatisfaction was unexpected. . . . Telephone access was by far the leading cause of patient dissatisfaction. Moreover, this problem was prominent in all departments and sites. The clinic's administrative team was aware of the phone problem, but has been unable to come up with solutions (short of adding expensive capacity). Therefore, telephone access seemed to be a good problem with which to test the application of 'industrial' quality management techniques."

This simple approach to "listening to the voice of the customer" produced an unexpected and valuable signal with which the project team could formulate its definition of the problem. Here is the initial statement of their goal: "To improve the entire process of obtaining medical information and/or an appointment by telephone in the family practice section of the medical center."

This project team, by the way, was later to discover that this initial problem statement was too broad to tackle. As they began to gather data, they were able to focus the problem on one particular part of the telephone system, namely, that involving access to the "medical information nurse." We will return to this story in Chapter Six.

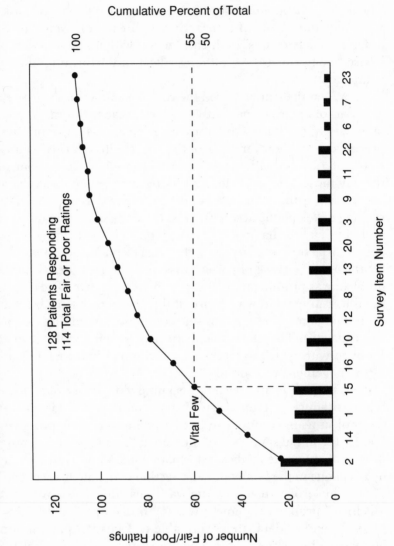

Exhibit 4.1. Reasons for Patient Dissatisfaction: A Pareto Diagram (Park Nicollet Project).

Exhibit 4.1. Reasons for Patient Dissatisfaction: A Pareto Diagram (Park Nicollet Project), Cont'd.

1. Ease of getting appointment
2. Ability to get through on phone
3. Attitude of phone receptionist
4. Attitude of clinic receptionist
5. Attitude of nurses
6. Willingness of staff to answer questions
7. Cleanliness of clinic
8. Ease of getting around in clinic
9. Attitude of lab personnel
10. Timely response to phone calls
11. Timely prescription refills
12. Billing process

13. Response to complaints
14. Communication about new services
15. Waiting time in reception area
16. Waiting time in examination room
17. Friendliness of doctor
18. Competence of doctor
19. Responsiveness of doctor
20. Amount of time spent with doctor
21. Concern shown by doctor
22. Information given you about diagnosis
23. Overall satisfaction

The team at Worcester Memorial Hospital used a more elaborate technique than a simple survey to derive project ideas from the external customers. They used a method called "Quality Function Deployment" (QFD) to decide which emergency department processes to work on.

As the Worcester team describes it, "QFD is a system for designing a product or service based on customer demands. . . . " The basic technique of QFD is simple: Create a two-dimensional matrix that relates what customers want (the key quality characteristics of a product or service) to the processes through which those key characteristics are produced. With careful inventory of customer needs (sometimes with importance weights attached), and "cross-indexing" those needs against processes, certain processes can be identified as especially important in shaping the customers' experiences. In its full form, QFD involves extensive technical analyses to derive optimal engineering specifications and to incorporate knowledge of the performance of competitors, but even a simple version like that used at Worcester Memorial Hospital can help set priorities in process improvement.

The Worcester Memorial Hospital team was able through a QFD matrix to identify three processes that were especially critical to patients' needs in the emergency room: "The response time of the laboratory department to emergency department patient orders; the level and quality of communications between emergency department staff and their patients; the process for admitting emergency department patients to an inpatient bed."

Because the team had selected problems specifically on the basis of their known relationships to customer needs, they could be more confident that improvement would pay off in the hospital's relationship with its patients.

Finding Problems Versus Finding Opportunities: The Limited Imagination of the External Customer

Surveys of external customers or examination of complaint files can be useful in setting priorities, but external customers are not always the best sources of truly innovative ideas for improvement. In surveys and complaints, customers tend not to spontaneously suggest clever improvements in processes, products, and services that, once offered, can truly delight them. To find these opportunities, special techniques, like focus groups, can be used to help customers free up their thinking about what would please and surprise them. In addition, organizations can tap other sources of ideas, such as their own employees and managers and studies of competitors and other industries.

This is especially true of what the Japanese quality expert Noritaki Kano calls "attractive quality" or "exciting quality." Kano suggests that the quality characteristics of a product or service can be roughly classified as "take-it-for-granted quality," "one-dimensional quality," or "attractive quality." "Take-it-for-granted quality" includes attributes that are routinely expected by customers, and the absence of which (but not the presence) will be noticed. Airline safety is one such attribute; it is hard to delight customers by claiming that one runs an airline that does not crash, but it is easy to disappoint them by evidence of poor safety.

"One-dimensional quality" involves attributes that have a more-or-less continuous relationship with customer satisfaction. In a hospital admitting office, for example, promptness of service is probably "one-dimensional." The speedier the service, the more satisfied the patient (assuming other features of quality remain the same).

"Attractive quality" delights customers in part because it is unexpected. Yet precisely because it is unexpected, it is difficult to get ideas for attractive quality from customers without specifically trying to do so. Few express mail customers, accustomed to delivery by the afternoon of the next day, might have spontaneously suggested next *morning* delivery. It took imagination and an intention to *exceed* expected quality levels for Federal Express to create a new industry standard: delivery by 10:30 A.M.

Organizations with mature quality improvement programs are very interested in ways to conceive and increase "attractive quality," thereby delighting those who depend on the organization. Such organizations search widely for ideas for improvement projects. They do ask their current customers, but they also welcome suggestions from employees, study their competitors, and look systematically outside their own areas and industries for clever new ideas.

The NDP project teams did not develop projects in "attractive quality." In most cases, they were oiling squeaky wheels. Their project ideas came from complaints, distress, and profiles of trouble as revealed in surveys and group brainstorming sessions. As a result, they tended to approach improvement as a matter of solving existing problems instead of imagining and realizing new opportunities. This is characteristic of early quality improvement efforts. In the first stages, problems are so widespread that it makes sense to start on the most irksome areas, "picking the low-hanging fruit," as some say. Later on, having solved some easier problems and having built skills in improvement methods, organizations and teams can be expected to think more easily in terms of new opportunities instead of old troubles.

Project Nominations from Internal Customers

Several of the project teams turned quickly and repeatedly to *internal* customers for ideas and for help in refining problem definitions. The team from Strong Memorial Hospital, for example, was concerned about patient flow in the emergency room, noting that patients there often waited an hour or more for simple care that took only minutes to administer.

Although the original topic came from interpretations of the needs of external customers, repeatedly the team sought out the staff of the emergency room and the hospital — with questionnaires, group meetings, and informal discussions — for help in localizing the issues. Which patients were involved in long waits? What steps in the process of patient care should be looked at most closely? What bothered the hospital staff the most about delays? The team was neither shy nor frightened to hear from the hospital's employees. They invented even more ways to listen, and, in their summary report, they wrote, "This project demonstrated to us that insights can be achieved by a fresh, systematic analysis of practices. The perspective of the 'internal customer' has been a particularly useful theme. This analysis led to a trial of a major change in the process of patient care not previously considered — the physician/nurse management team (which was used to evaluate and triage patients in the emergency room)."

The understanding achieved at Strong Memorial Hospital came directly from the open relationships the team developed with internal customers in the processes of emergency room care. They made partners of their customers.

Other Ways to Select Projects: Criterion Matrices and Analyzing the Cost of Poor Quality

Other devices were used by the NDP teams for choosing among ideas for projects. The Harvard Community Health Plan team selected its topic — variation in use of ultrasound tests — partly by using a *criterion matrix* of desired characteristics for a proposed topic. For example, they decided that a project would be more likely to succeed if it tackled a clinical issue that occurred *frequently,* that involved *substantial cost,* for which there was existing evidence of *variation in practice,* and for which *data were easily available.* The team rated each proposed topic on these criteria and selected ultrasonography as overall the best candidate for further work.

Lists of criteria for selecting improvement projects exist in many standard textbooks of quality improvement. Beyond those employed by the Harvard Community Health Plan team, other common criteria for selecting good improvement projects include, for example:

- Avoid working on processes for which change is currently planned or already underway.
- Choose processes that managers and employees believe need to be improved.
- Choose processes that are clearly defined — ones with clear starting and ending points.
- Choose processes that have short "cycle times," so that data are readily available and the effects of interventions easier to study.

Another approach to selecting projects involves assessing the "cost of poor quality" — that is, estimating how much is currently being lost in waste, rework, unreliability, decreased morale, customer disaffection, and the many other ways in which quality problems erode efficiency. The Massachusetts General Hospital team had such an estimate in mind when it selected accuracy of Medicare billing as its initial NDP topic. The team constructed a specific dollar estimate of direct cash flow losses, and noted further that that figure certainly underestimated the full cost of poor quality: "If the combined problems of inaccurate and delayed billing of Medicare services persisted, the cost to Massachusetts General Hospital of delayed cash flow would total approximately $360,000 per year. An added cost is that for the additional personnel devoted to correcting inaccuracies and re-billing rejected claims. All rejected claims must be rebilled manually by hospital personnel and processed manually by Medicare. This again slows the process and increases the probability of making a second error. Finally, this volume of rejections causes significant confusion and unpredictability within the system. Reducing the confusion and improving the predictability of payment and cash flow could only enhance our financial stability."

Specific analyses like this of the cost of poor quality can help motivate both teams and organizational leaders toward process improvement. It is important, however, to keep in mind that direct cost control is only one among the many benefits that accrue to organizations that learn how to improve their quality continuously. Too much emphasis on cost containment can divert energy from the more central goal of improving processes. When processes are made better, total costs usually fall. However, starting with the question "What costs can we reduce?" can lead teams astray, away from process improvement and into mere budget cutting.

Key Principles in Constructing a Sound Problem Statement

Sound problem statements (some call them "opportunity statements") for teams can take many forms, but adhering to a few key principles can help. Statements that conform to the following guidelines lessen the probability of rework, because they reduce the likelihood that a team will discover that it has set to work on "the wrong question."

Principle 1: The Problem Statement Should Reflect Shared Values and a Clear Purpose.   It is difficult to set about improving a process unless the purpose of the process is clearly understood. If the purpose is unclear, then the word *improvement* is essentially undefined. This apparently simple point can create some difficulties for improvement teams. Trying to state the team's purpose clearly can involve some difficult negotiations and can include a few surprises at the start.

At the Park Nicollet Medical Center, for example, a team that turned its attention to "improving urgent care access" for patients soon discovered that team members disagreed about what "improvement" meant. For some team members, "improved" access implied more protection of the physicians from medically trivial unscheduled encounters with patients. For other team members, "improved" access meant better availability of immediate appointments for patients who requested them.

Obviously, trouble is in store for a team that tries to continue its work without uncovering and, in one way or another, resolving such differences. The team needs skills in uncovering such disagreements and working toward consensus. It may need to appeal to a higher organizational authority to better define what the purpose of the process should be in light of the organization's overall goals. Sometimes, happily, the team can discover so-called "win-win" options, in which revising a process can serve everyone's interests better, in effect abolishing the apparent conflict in aims.

It is a tough job for the leader of a team to find ways to build bridges among team members, so that the purpose of the team is clear and acceptable to all. But it is not a job that can be safely neglected. In fact, many experts on quality management urge that team leaders and facilitators receive specific, focused training on group process skills such as leading discussions, brainstorming, and conflict resolution in groups.

Principle 2: The Problem Statement Should Not Mention Either Causes or Remedies.   A second common issue in defining the problem is the way in which preconceptions can impede the gathering of new knowledge. When a problem has existed

for a long time, *almost everyone* can feel sure that they know why
the problem exists and what "they" (that is, someone else) should
do about it. The answer is "obvious."

The group at Evanston Hospital confronted this issue
almost immediately. The ambulatory surgery program at that
hospital had grown from 23 percent of all operations to 40 percent between 1985 and 1987, with a daily volume increase of
81 percent. Problems were appearing in patient flow; it seemed
that not enough staff were available to process patients and delays in surgery were increasingly common. The cause seemed
obvious; as the team's report puts it, "Because several staff in
the ambulatory surgery program had expressed concern about
increased volume, this was initially the presumed primary cause
for delays in the operating room."

Such a prior belief is common, but what happened next
was not. Instead of taking the usual steps of simply advocating
more staff, perhaps armed with some hastily collected numbers
to "prove" that more staff were needed, the team turned to a
scientific question: "Can we, by understanding the process of
patient flow in the ambulatory surgery unit, *verify* that staffing
deficiencies are causing delay? Or, can we uncover other root
causes of delay that can be remedied in other ways?"

In Chapter Six, we will follow in detail the "diagnostic
journey" that this team took as it searched for root causes of
delay. As it turned out, the major causes of delay had little to
do with either volume or staffing ratios. Deficiencies in the flow
of preoperative information, for example, were one key, and
had nothing to do with case volume.

One quality expert has gone so far as to say that, in quality
improvement efforts, "more staff," "more space," and "more
money" almost never turn out to be the best remedies. At Evanston Hospital, the *problem* was delay in surgery. One hypothesis about the *cause* of the problem was "not enough staff"; but,
in the method of quality improvement, *all* sound hypotheses must
be considered and tested. If a team starts out with a particular
remedy in mind by, for example, defining "the problem" as "not
enough staff," it may never get to understand the process and
the real causes of flaw. "More staff" at Evanston Hospital would

have been only a Band-Aid, and a costly one, covering up the true process flaws: waste, rework, and unnecessary complexity. To begin a truly open-minded journey toward discovery of root causes requires a special degree of trust. In classically managed organizations, the fight for more resources is so familiar that it can feel naive and even dangerous to let go, even temporarily, of the battle, and to ask instead if a better process can be designed without more staff, more space, or more money — perhaps with even less.

The guidelines for a sound problem statement include avoidance of suggesting blame ("they do it to us"), cause ("this is why the defects happen"), or solutions ("we need a new computer") in the problem statement. Here is a problem statement doomed from the start: "Patients are waiting too long because, without a computerized scheduling system, we have too few staff to register them correctly." Another example that will cause trouble: "Evaluation of ectopic pregnancies is too often delayed because the laboratory loses initial blood specimens or fails to give us stat results fast enough." Better versions avoid blaming, stating causes, or suggesting remedies: "Delays in patient registration are frustrating to the patients, and lead to inefficient use of the time of clinical staff." Or: "More rapid diagnostic management of patients with possible ectopic pregnancies would increase patient safety and improve their clinical outcomes."

Principle 3: The Problem Statement Should Define Problems and Processes of Manageable Size. The team from the Kaiser-Permanente Medical Care Program of Northern California knew from the start what it wanted to work on; it was a problem that surfaced almost immediately in a group brainstorming session. They wrote, "When a medical center patient appears for follow-up care after hospital emergency treatment, and the emergency department record is not at hand, the quality of care can be affected."

The Kaiser-Permanente care system consists of fourteen medical centers, each with a hospital, an emergency room, and an adjoining ambulatory care facility, as well as several satellite medical office buildings affiliated with a medical center but located in a different city or area. Kaiser-Permanente patients are members of a particular group practice, which may be in a satellite medical office building, but at special times, like nights or weekends or in severe emergencies, they may seek care in an emergency room at a medical center. Kaiser-Permanente physicians and staff knew that, when a patient received emergency care, the record of that care often did not reach the patient's "home" physician, which disrupted the continuity of care.

In the way it approached defining the problem, the Kaiser-Permanente team illustrated one of the key principles in that step of problem solving, namely, "define a problem of manageable size": "The problem originally selected by the Kaiser-Permanente Medical Care Program for the National Demonstration Project was the timely transfer of clinical data from medical centers to their satellite medical office buildings. After due consideration, the scope of the issue was recognized to be too broad. Major progress in selection occurred when the project was narrowed. It was limited to one medical center, the Kaiser-Permanente Santa Clara Medical Center (SCL) with its two satellites, Milpitas (MIL) and Sunnyvale (SUN). Furthermore, the group assembled to work on the issue (the physician-in-chief, physicians-in-charge, facility administrators, and selected department heads from SCL, SUN, and MIL) narrowed it to one particular area of clinical information transfer which was especially bothersome to staff and patients: 'the timely transfer of appropriate emergency department clinical data from SCL to its two satellites, MIL and SUN.'"

The Kaiser-Permanente team reports "major progress" when they "narrowed" the problem they were to tackle. Such "narrowing" is vital to the success of quality improvement efforts. How did they narrow the problem? In several ways. They bounded it *geographically* (to SCL, MIL, and SUN, as opposed to the whole organization); they restricted it to a particular *clinical area* (emergency department records, instead of all medical center data); and they focused on a particular *dimension of quality* or a single *key quality characteristic* (timeliness of data transfer, instead of data quality, accuracy, legibility, clinical appropriateness, or some large set of desired outputs).

Many strategies for narrowing the problem are possible, of course. Beyond those used by Kaiser-Permanente, for example, such strategies can include choosing a particular *time interval* to work on (such as "afternoon telephone response" instead of simply "telephone response"), a particular *diagnosis* or *type of clinical care* (such as "asthma visits" or "cataract surgery" instead of "same-day visits" or "surgery"), or a particular *customer group* ("giving medication instructions to the elderly" instead of "instructing patients about medication").

Few project teams concluded, in the end, that they had chosen too small a problem. Several lamented that what seemed tractable at the start turned out to be far too large a problem for a single team to work on. Quality improvement wins wars through many small battles; it seeks cumulative results, not single, dramatic victories.

Principle 4: The Problem Statement Should, If Possible, Mention Measurable Characteristics.   Not all characteristics of quality are easy to measure, but many are. When possible, the problem definition itself should imply measurements through which the improvement effort can be monitored.

Using this principle, it is better to begin with an effort "to improve the timeliness and legibility of preliminary X-ray reports to emergency room physicians" than it is to try "to improve X-ray service to emergency room physicians." The former problem statement implies quantifiable features of the X-ray reporting process, the latter does not. As it tried to localize the problem and to monitor gains, a team with the former statement in its charter would know that it should measure time intervals and find a way to score the legibility of reports. A team starting with the latter statement would have trouble beginning its diagnostic efforts and, in the end, trouble knowing whether improvement had occurred.

Principle 5: The Problem Statement Should Be Refined as Process Knowledge Is Gained.   Getting a clear statement of the problem is essential to effective teamwork, but revisiting and revising the statement is also a sign of a healthy team. Problem definition in quality improvement is more like an ascending spiral than a single task. In its first steps, the team tries its best to state a problem clearly. As it gains knowledge of the processes involved, it may (and usually does) return to the problem statement more than once, revising and changing it—focusing it—in light of its learning.

The Massachusetts Respiratory Hospital team began with one problem and then changed its agenda based on deeper knowledge. Their initial concern was the cost and discontinuity in care that resulted from the hospital's use of "agency nurses"—that is, part-time, contract nurses who were called in for brief periods of work to supplement the salaried nurse staff of the hospital. The team's first problem statement was this: "How could Massachusetts Respiratory Hospital reduce dependence on agency nurses, improve the morale of the existing staff, and, most importantly, improve the quality of care delivered to Massachusetts Respiratory Hospital patients?"

This team began by trying to understand the process through which agency nurses were hired, and the team's initial diagram of the process *began* with the assumption that an agency nurse was needed. Quickly, the team refocused on the prior issue: why agency nurses were needed in the first place. This led them to study nursing staff turnover, and to a question that became their new problem statement: "Why are staff nurses leaving Massachusetts Respiratory Hospital?" In the team's subsequent work, agency nursing was not even mentioned; data were collected instead on staff nurse separations and their underlying causes.

Another example of refining a problem statement appears in the work of the team from Boston's Children's Hospital. The initial problem selected by the team there was delay in the process of transporting critically ill infants from outlying hospitals to the tertiary care center at Children's Hospital. Transport began with a request from an outlying hospital, following which a transport team was assembled at Children's Hospital and sent to the outlying hospital. There, the patient was evaluated, placed in an ambulance, and taken to Children's Hospital under medical supervision. The team was concerned about " . . . complaints that the transport often takes too long to arrive, too long to stabilize the patient, and pays too little attention to physician/community hospital relations."

After collecting data on actual transport times, the team was able to redefine their project. Although they had suspected at the outset that delays en route and at the outlying hospital were severe, the actual data showed that the "in-house" time (the time spent preparing the transport team to leave from Children's Hospital to travel to the outlying facility) was the major source of delay. With such process knowledge, a more focused problem statement was possible: "To reduce the in-house time between the call for transport and the dispatch of the transport team."

The spiral of problem definition led to a clearer agenda for process improvement and a new, refined problem statement.

Conclusions

The experience of the NDP teams offers guidance for sound problem definition. The lessons they learned are several:

- Search widely among customers, both external and internal, for ideas for improvement projects.
- Remain open-minded about causes and remedies, and, in particular, do not cling fearfully to the hypotheses that more staff, more space, or more money must be the best solution.
- Formulate crisp, clear statements of the opportunity for improvement, and avoid in those statements implications of blame, hypotheses of cause, or suggestions of remedy.
- Narrow the problem scope using sensible boundaries of geography, diagnosis, quality dimension, and whatever else makes sense.
- Finally, revisit the problem statement often, and revise it as your understanding increases about the processes underlying the symptoms.

The NDP teams tackled a wide assortment of problems, for example:

- At Butterworth Hospital, the respiratory therapy department wanted to increase their capability to satisfy requests for respiratory therapy services: The demand exceeded their capacity.
- At Massachusetts General Hospital, a high proportion of bills to Medicare were being returned unpaid because the bill was incorrect.
- At Park Nicollet Medical Center, patients were complaining about telephone access in a family practice unit.
- At Children's Hospital, the time taken to fetch critically ill infants needing transport from outlying hospitals seemed too long.
- At three hospitals — University of Michigan Hospitals, North Carolina Memorial Hospital, and Boston's Beth Israel Hospital — delayed discharge of patients was tying up rooms and frustrating staff and patients.
- At Harvard Community Health Plan, variation among clinical units in their use of ultrasonography in pregnant women seemed excessive.

There was, in short, no end to the problems available to work on. In many cases, the problems were chronic; they were well known and, as one project team put it, "had eluded solution for decades." Now, with the quality improvement method, these problems were to be "scheduled for solution."

5

Organizing Quality Improvement Teams

Why a Team?

Almost all modern models of quality improvement use teams. The legendary companies in quality management—Toyota, Florida Power and Light, Honda, Xerox—report that they have hundreds or even thousands of project teams in place at any particular time. In fact, teams are so pervasive as a device in quality improvement that some newcomers mistakenly conclude that employee teams, or "quality circles," are *all there is to it.*

In fact, quality improvement involves a great deal more than teams and teamwork. In fully mature quality management organizations, the methods of improvement—defining the problem, formulating hypotheses, collecting data, and so forth— are visible everywhere and all the time. There is no longer a crisp distinction between quality improvement work and the rest of work. Nonetheless, beyond this pervasive "quality improvement in daily worklife," employees also continue to serve regularly on specially created cross-functional project teams.

Quality improvement teams help in several ways. First, they facilitate dialogue, understanding, and knowledge of processes that cross formal departmental boundaries. Understanding a process often requires that people from different staff areas, and people from different hierarchical levels, think together—

people who, without a team, might never meet each other. These special opportunities to work together are necessary simply because no single person occupies a perch from which the whole process is visible, and yet it is *precisely* the *whole process* that is the object of improvement. When people work hard at improving only their own, visible, local segment of a process, the result may be that, while their segment is made better, the process as a whole is made worse.

Industrial engineers call such myopic improvement "suboptimization." One common example of suboptimization occurs when a local group checks the work of others, either because they do not trust the others, or because they do not know what forms of checking have already occurred. This adds waste, redundancy, and complexity to a process, even though it feels better to the local group. Teams offer an opportunity to improve the whole process, instead of suboptimizing segments of it.

Second, teams provide a useful setting for formal training of employees in quality improvement tools such as process flow analysis, data collection, and histograms. For many people, the best time to learn such tools is when they have a need to use them at a specific point in an improvement project. The team meeting can be an efficient place to deliver "just-in-time" training in the methods as they are used.

Third, teams and well-run team meetings can help keep projects on schedule and moving along. The team can create deadlines, set agendas, and help its members feel both shared enthusiasm and mutual obligations. Charging a team to carry out an assignment in process improvement formally declares a problem "scheduled for solution," and celebrating the accomplishments of a team is a clear way to record and memorialize achievements in the quality improvement process.

Teams in the National Demonstration Project

A few of the original NDP participants never reached the stage of designing a project, but every one that went so far as to begin work on a process did so with a quality improvement team. Some set up a classical "quality council" — that is, a leadership group of executives who then charged a lower-level cross-functional team to work on a specific problem. Strong Memorial Hospital, for example, formed an "advisory group" containing senior executives, including the president of the hospital, along with teams reporting regularly to the advisory group as they tried to improve patient flow in the emergency room. Kaiser-Permanente Medical Care Program also used a two-tiered structure: a steering committee of senior managers, and a working group of middle-level managers, supervisors, and front-line staff.

In other cases, as part of this initial organizational experiment, executives joined directly with lower-level employees in the work of an improvement team. The Evanston Hospital team, which worked on ambulatory surgery delays, *included* the chief executive officer of Evanston Hospital, the senior vice president, and the assistant to the president, as well as nurses and coordinators from the clinical areas involved. The same profile of participation occurred at Park Nicollet Medical Center. Team members at the Worcester Memorial Hospital (where the task was improving emergency room services) included, interestingly, several members of the board of trustees.

The value of the visible participation of the executives, whether as members of teams or of the steering committees, was stressed repeatedly in the project reports. Butterworth Hospital, for example, reported the following: "One of the main reasons for the project's successes was top management's initial 'buy in.' The vice president responsible for the respiratory care department attended every meeting of the quality improvement task force. This participation eased implementation of the team's solutions. Some decisions which historically had required many reviews were acted on directly."

Similarly, the Massachusetts General Hospital report states: "Without question, the most instrumental factor in the success in reducing billing inaccuracies and analyzing billing delays has been the commitment from high levels of the organization to solve the problem. This commitment has come not only from administration, but also from key representatives of the medical staff. As a result of this support, the interdepartmental project team and its staff resources have been able to bring diverse areas of knowledge and expertise to focus on a difficult issue that typically crosses departmental and functional lines of communication and authority."

NDP project teams ranged in size from two to twenty members, with a median of nine. Most met weekly or every other week for several months, and several used a "subcommittee" structure to tackle specific elements of the processes they were studying. At Worcester Memorial Hospital, for example, having identified three key processes in the emergency room (laboratory test ordering, communication with patients and families, and transfer from the emergency room to an acute inpatient bed), the team designated one subgroup to work on each. Of the eighteen teams submitting specific reports, fourteen included at least one physician.

No clear pattern emerged regarding the relationship between team structures and team effectiveness. Among the most successful projects one finds both large teams and small ones and both "two-tiered" structures (a council or steering group plus working groups) and "single-tiered" structures. The successful projects all do have one thing in common, however: the visible presence of top organizational leaders in a regular role — either in reviewing the teams' progress or in actually participating on a team. There appears to be no effective substitute for the time of top leaders, at least in the early stages of the quality improvement effort. Other important ingredients in sound teamwork included regularity of meetings, adequate time devoted to team training, and open dialogue among team members.

Extending Horizons

In the NDP team reports, testimonials abound to the value of simply *having* a team, even before the statistical methods of process improvement were used. The common theme is the power of the cross-functional teams to extend the horizons of managers and employees who previously understood only their own local part of the processes involved.

The Butterworth Hospital team, brought together to improve the ability of the respiratory therapy department to satisfy clinicians' requests for respiratory care, included the vice president of the hospital, the director of the respiratory care department, respiratory care staff members from different roles and levels, and representatives (a nurse and a unit secretary) from some clinical areas served. The team reported: "Because of the team-oriented problem-solving atmosphere that was established early in the task force, an interesting situation was observed at the first meeting. The discussion centered around the processes by which respiratory care was ordered in the hospital. The team noticed a significant difference between how this process was working and how it was designed to work. The process differed not only between the nursing division staff and the respiratory care staff, but also between respiratory care groups. This lack of a common process was restricting availability of equipment and limiting our ability to provide service."

This discovery of a "significant difference between how this process was working and how it was designed to work" is not unique to Butterworth Hospital. It is the almost universal discovery of process improvement teams who sit together to document, perhaps for the first time, how a "familiar" work process is actually conducted. "Aha," they all say, "we never knew that before." All it took was enough knowledge in one room at one time along with a tool as simple as the process flow diagram.

The Massachusetts General Hospital report mentions a related revelation that comes first from the mere existence of a team: the clarification of internal customer-supplier relationships. The problem at issue was how to generate an accurate and prompt bill to Medicare for hospital services; inaccurate bills were being returned frequently without payment: "The cooperative team approach toward quality improvement has forged common understanding among specialists. Physicians on the team have learned how their actions impact admitting and medical records, and these departments in turn have grown to understand how their actions impact billing. This common understanding has only strengthened what was from the beginning a strong commitment to reducing defects and encouraging progress toward quality improvement in this area."

A related benefit of teamwork was in a few cases the team's clarification of "ownership" of a key process. For example, the Kaiser-Permanente group (working on timely transfer of emergency room records to satellite medical office buildings) wrote, "An important element fell into place when one of the members of the working group declared 'ownership' of the (record transfer) process." Complex processes, crossing departmental and organizational boundaries, often lack a single manager who can keep the whole process in mind. The "process owner" is an individual who can serve as organizational eyes and ears on the whole process (as it is experienced by the customer, not as it is divided up by the organization), and can exercise the authority to convene and coordinate improvement and quality control efforts. When a process owner is identified, improvement has a better chance.

Leading Teams

Leading a team is a challenge for which few people have been specifically trained. A complete training program in quality management must include team leadership skills. Having had some prior training, a few NDP team leaders did employ specific techniques for helping groups think together more effectively. The "nominal group method" for generating a list of ideas and "multivoting" for prioritizing the ideas both appear in the work of the Harvard Community Health Plan group. Formal "brainstorming," which has a particular set of rules for group process, was used at Butterworth Hospital and Massachusetts Respiratory Hospital.

In the project reports, there is a striking *lack* of comment on formal group leadership techniques, suggesting either that these techniques were not necessary at the early stage of work in the NDP or that they are unfamiliar to those who worked in and with the teams. The experience of others in project teamwork suggests that those who begin to use quality improvement methods widely would benefit from specific instruction in brainstorming, multivoting, nominal group process, conflict resolution, meeting planning, and a few other specific small-group leadership techniques.

A positive image of good group process emerges in a comment from the Kaiser-Permanente report: "The group members were motivated in their interactions with the issue and with each other, and skillful in their communications and interpersonal relationships. Of note was the fact that no one dominated the work sessions, and members were able to provide information and to express their views clearly and succinctly."

Perhaps this was a group of extraordinarily collaborative people. However, it is also likely that this group had the benefit of a leader skilled in facilitating dialogue, disclosure, and trust.

Helping Teams

Behind every project team in the NDP was an experienced quality management professional donating his or her time to help introduce a method for improvement in a health care organization. They are a remarkably quiet bunch in the actual project reports. It appears that they were, from the start, intent on teaching people to fish instead of delivering fish to them. Between the lines, one hears their guiding voices:

> It was suggested that a process flow diagram would help us understand the process further.

> We gained insight when our quality advisor suggested displaying data in an hour-by-hour control chart.

> At our first meeting, the hospital teams and consultants decided that Delphi-type surveys would be undertaken to ask staff about the internal and external causes of delayed discharges.

Subtly, the simple tools of quality improvement appear in the work of the teams: cause-and-effect diagrams, histograms, control charts, Pareto charts, scatterplots, and clever ways to collect and stratify data.

The lesson is that expertise in quality improvement involves the ability to help others gain skills in understanding processes, not just in knowing how to analyze and improve processes as a visiting fire fighter. If quality improvement involved calling in experts, we could simply hire engineers and be done with it. The real development of organizationwide capabilities in quality improvement is slower but in the end immensely more powerful. For many employees, participation in a quality improvement team is their first introduction to the skills of process improvement that will, from then on, be part of their daily work.

6

The Diagnostic Journey

If we think of quality improvement itself as a process consisting of *defining the problem, making the diagnosis, administering the remedy,* and *holding the gains,* then we may ask, as we may of any process: What does each step receive from the previous step — its supplier — and provide to the next step — its customer? We have seen how the teams in the National Demonstration Project arrived at a statement of the problem they would be focusing on. Using the process described and analyzed in Chapter Four, each group "supplied" a clear, well-informed problem statement that could then serve as the starting point for the next step: making the diagnosis.

As we will see, the "diagnostic journey" is in many cases a long and tortuous one; complicated issues often underlie the simplest diagnostic questions. Quality improvement has its own "black bag" of many specialized instruments — process flow diagrams, histograms, Pareto diagrams, Ishikawa diagrams, and more — for making the diagnosis (these tools are described in detail in Resource B). Despite the many new terms and tools introduced in the diagnostic enterprise, however, making the diagnosis is a conceptually simple procedure. It consists of two basic steps:

1. Defining and understanding the existing process.
2. Analyzing the existing process to determine where the flaws — and thus the opportunities for improvement — lie.

Despite the variety of problems and areas of health care tackled by the teams in the NDP in the course of their diagnostic journeys, we will see that their experiences have much in common. The departure point is a well-framed problem statement. The group begins the diagnostic journey by making a map of the process as it currently exists, continues by analyzing the process to generate hypotheses about possible flaws, and then moves to gathering data to test whether *those* particular flaws exist at *those* particular points in the process. Their work is an exact analogue of the scientific method used in modern research: ask a question, formulate hypotheses, and then, using data, seek to confirm, reject, or modify the hypotheses.

By the end of the diagnostic journey, a project team should be able to answer the following questions: "What goes wrong?" "Where?" and "How do we know?" The answers to these questions, in turn, are key inputs to the next step—the remedial journey—which has its own agenda for hypothesis generation ("What might *help* here?") and testing ("Does the remedy *work*?").

This chapter analyzes the diagnostic journeys of several project teams, using them to demonstrate three key stages of the journey: first, understanding the existing process; second, generating and testing hypotheses about where and why the process is flawed; and third, displaying and understanding data.

Defining and Understanding the Existing Process: Two Case Studies

In quality improvement efforts it is always helpful to ask, "what is the process that we intend to improve?" Defining existing processes as clearly as possible is a key step in the work of a team, as two specific cases from the NDP illustrate.

Kaiser-Permanente.   The experience of the team at the Kaiser-Permanente Medical Care Program in Northern California shows the two-step nature of diagnosing the problem. The Kaiser-Permanente team had identified an apparently simple procedural problem that was affecting the quality of care in a variety of ways: When a patient appeared for a follow-up ap-

pointment at one of the Kaiser-Permanente medical office buildings subsequent to receiving hospital emergency treatment, the
patient's emergency records were frequently unavailable. As we
saw in Chapter Four, the group wisely chose to narrow the scope
of its inquiry, in the words of its carefully articulated problem
statement, to "the timely transfer of appropriate emergency
department clinical data from the Santa Clara Medical Center
to its two satellites, [the medical office buildings in] Milpitas
and Sunnyvale."

The Kaiser-Permanente team began to tackle the problem by *examining the existing process* for transferring emergency
treatment data to the medical office building at which the patient received subsequent treatment. To accomplish this, they
used a basic tool of quality improvement, the *process flow diagram.* (For a complete discussion, see Resource B.) The process
flow diagram is useful in many ways. First, it converts what
may seem like a vague, complicated collection of events into
a graphic display of a clear, visible series of steps. More important, the very exercise of creating the flow diagram forces the
group to see a "problem" in terms of a process, and it highlights
the various inefficiencies and obstructions that may lie within
it. The flow diagram helps people recognize that, underlying
even the most haphazard, unplanned collection of events in
work, there *is* a process. A process does not have to be efficient,
or well conceived, or even *intentional;* it is merely the way work
is done. Forcing oneself to commit to paper a description of the
existing process—becoming aware of it *as* a process—is an important step toward improving quality.

The act of creating the process flow diagram was particularly revealing in the Kaiser-Permanente case. Based on their
collective perceptions of what happened to a patient's medical
record from the time of entering the emergency room to the
follow-up office visit, the members of the Kaiser-Permanente
team created the flow diagram displayed in Exhibit 6.1.

The diagram shows the following steps: When the patient
arrives in the emergency room, the receptionist asks for his or
her "home facility." Depending on the answer—MIL (Milpitas),
SUN (Sunnyvale), or SCL (Santa Clara)—the receptionist tags

Exhibit 6.1. Initial Description of Record Transfer Process:
A Process Flow Diagram (Kaiser-Permanente Project).

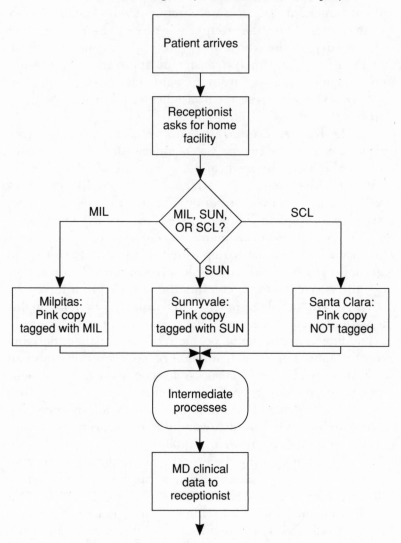

Exhibit 6.1. Initial Description of Record Transfer Process:
A Process Flow Diagram (Kaiser-Permanente Project), Cont'd.

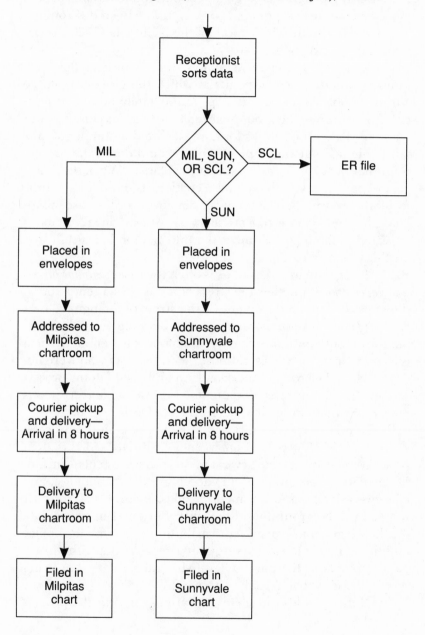

the pink copy of the patient's record, indicating the home facility. After the patient's emergency room treatment, clinical data are given to the receptionist, sorted, and delivered through a series of steps to the chart room of the facility at which the patient receives follow-up care.

As the team began its analysis of the process flow diagram to identify specific points at which the process could go wrong, problems at various steps immediately became apparent. For example, the group realized that at the apparently simple step, "Receptionist asks for home facility," a number of mistakes might occur, any one of which would derail the process from the start. As the group's report explains: "When the emergency room was very busy, the receptionists did not have time to get the information. Patients under stress, or because of language barriers, gave erroneous answers. At least one receptionist expected patients to volunteer the information because a sign on the wall asked that they do so."

The group found that, as is often the case, *when the process was under stress* — whether the stress of a busy emergency room, the stress of a patient in pain, or the stress of a language barrier — *it failed to work as it was designed.* Obtaining accurate information about the home facility might be easy enough when the emergency room was not busy, with patients who were not distracted and who could speak and read English; but the process was meant to work for *all* patients at *all* times, and as it was presently functioning, it was clearly inadequate to do so.

Another problem surfaced at a later step in the process: the sorting of all copies of emergency visit data. At this step, copies were distributed to several in-house departments — including pediatrics, obstetrics and gynecology, ophthalmology, and allergy — as well as to the medical office buildings. On closer inspection, the group found that distribution of in-house data was being given priority over distribution to the medical office buildings (in the language of quality improvement, the internal customers of the Santa Clara Medical Center were being served before the external customers).

Not only were problems at various steps in the process

immediately apparent; the team members were surprised to find that the *actual* process was in fact far more complicated than they had thought it to be. As they came to a clearer and clearer understanding of the process, the group put the original flow diagram through a series of revisions. Exhibit 6.2 is a later version of the same process represented in Exhibit 6.1. It indicates, for example, that (1) the receptionist may or may not ask for home facility and shows how the process proceeds in each case. Next, it reflects that (2) even if the receptionist does ask for home facility, the patient may or may not provide an answer, and indicates what happens in each case; later, (3) it more accurately reflects the path information takes from the emergency room to the site of follow-up care.

Not only did drawing the flow diagram help the team discover the actual process, it also made them realize in practice what they had heard of in theory: *the importance of customer-supplier relationships.* In the case of proper transfer of patient records, that meant recognizing that at each step along the way, there is a "customer" and a "supplier" and that the job of the supplier is to pass on to the customer *what,* and *only what,* he or she needs. The team reported: "The analytic process revealed unnecessary delivery of information to some departments and satellites, and inadequate delivery to others. During this process of revision, the actual information needs of the clinical departments and of the medical office buildings (all internal customers) were clarified and reclarified."

In the process flow diagram (Exhibit 6.2), for example, the receptionist is the *supplier,* whose job it is to determine accurately the site for follow-up care for every patient treated in the emergency room and to pass that information on to the next step along the way. The very exercise of creating the flow diagram helped clinical departments and medical office buildings clarify their roles and requirements as *customers;* what information did they need and what information was unnecessary? This, in turn, helped the emergency room understand its responsibility as *supplier* of information necessary for subsequent treatment of the patient.

Exhibit 6.2. Revised Description of Record Transfer Process:
A Process Flow Diagram (Kaiser-Permanente Project).

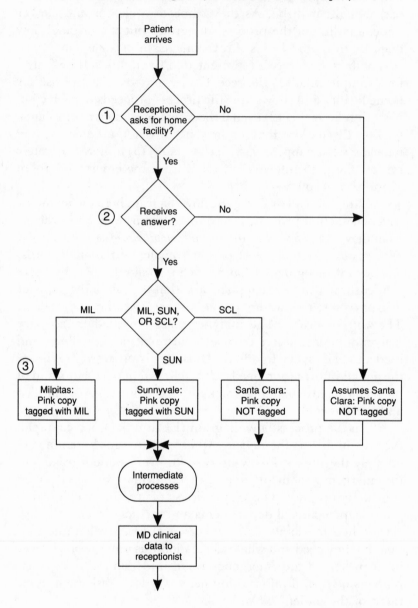

Exhibit 6.2. Revised Description of Record Transfer Process:
A Process Flow Diagram (Kaiser-Permanente Project), Cont'd.

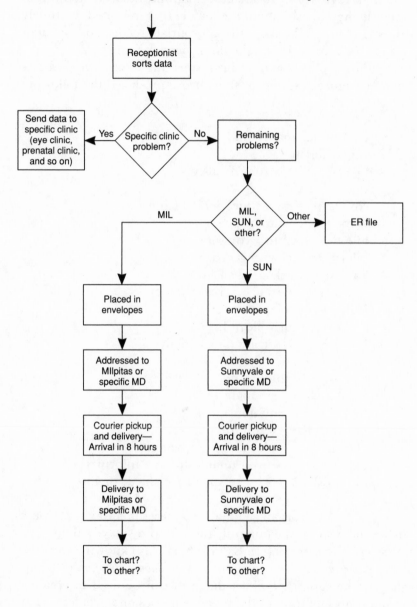

Once the Kaiser-Permanente team had created, analyzed, and then revised its process flow diagram, the next step was to generate hypotheses about the factors that inhibited the timely transfer of hospital data to the appropriate medical office building. Where and why might the process be failing?

The group began by brainstorming a list of hypotheses among themselves, and in short order produced the following list.

File lost in mailroom
Copy illegible
File sorted to wrong facility
White tag not used
No clarified procedure for labeling
Wrong information given
File delivered to wrong location
File sorted in wrong order
Patient not asked in effective way
File sent to wrong address
Duplicate copies received
Original record illegible
File sorted to wrong department
No copy made
Patient information not asked for
Duplicate copies made
Labeling information incomplete
Patient changes mind later
Document misplaced before being labeled
Patient refuses or is unable to give information
File mishandled by recipient, misfiled, or lost

In order to organize their hypotheses in a way that would make them more meaningful, the group displayed them in a *cause-and-effect diagram* (see Exhibit 6.3). Also known as an *Ishikawa diagram* (after its inventor) or a *fishbone diagram* (after its shape), the cause-and-effect diagram can be used to create a visual representation of the possible causes of a problem. (For a complete discussion, see Resource B.)

Exhibit 6.3. Cause-and-Effect Diagram for Timely Transfer of Emergency
Room Records to Satellite Medical Office Building (Kaiser-Permanente Project).

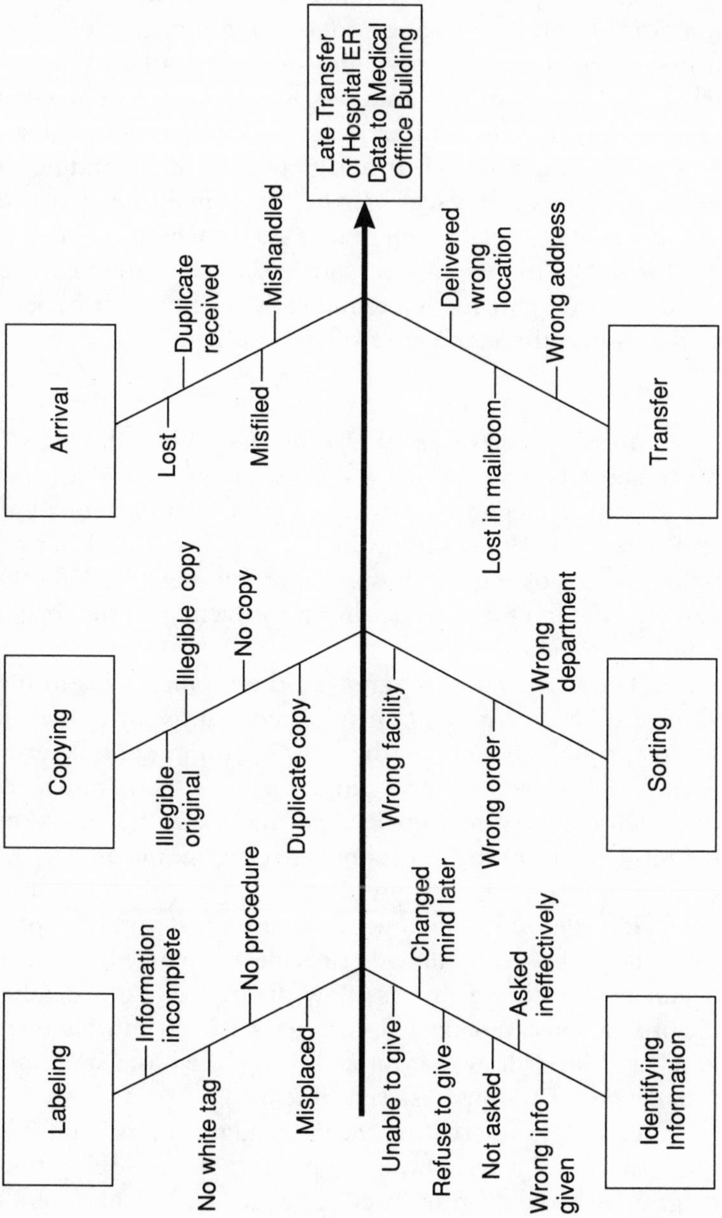

The diagram identifies six major possible points at which the process could go wrong—identifying information, sorting, transfer, labeling, copying, and arrival—and within each of these, a number of explanations for each particular error.

What had the Kaiser-Permanente team learned so far? First, the team had a clear and detailed understanding of the existing process, and second, they had analyzed that process and developed specific hypotheses about where it was flawed. At this point, the team was ready to move to the next step in the diagnostic journey: systematically testing their hypotheses to determine the root cause of the problem.

Massachusetts General Hospital.   When the team from Massachusetts General Hospital chose to tackle its Medicare billing system, it began by calculating the "cost of poor quality," and determined that the problems of delayed and inaccurate billing were costing the hospital approximately $360,000 per year. In the language of quality improvement, they began by clearly "proving the need."

The first step in diagnosing the problem was to inspect all of the Medicare inpatient rejected claims for a one-month sample, collecting data on the most common reasons for rejection. At this stage, the team did not have to spend much energy documenting the symptoms, as was the case with Kaiser-Permanente; the reasons for rejection were clearly indicated by Medicare, and required only simple tabulation (see Exhibit 6.4).

In order to understand at what points, and for what reasons, the process was failing to provide acceptable bills, the team began by creating a process flow diagram of steps leading to the production of a patient's bill. They started with what is known as a "high-level" flow diagram, showing the basic steps and the broad flow of the process (Exhibit 6.5).

Once again, creating the flow diagram was helpful to the group in many ways: "Both the process of developing the flow diagram and the diagram itself enhanced each department's understanding of internal customer-supplier relationships—that is, how one area affects the next in the production of a 'clean bill.'

Exhibit 6.4. Common Reasons for Rejection, 10/29/87–11/20/87
(Massachusetts General Hospital Project).

Reasons for Rejection	No. of Claims	Percent of Claims
Invalid/Missing HIC No.	32	20.0
Medicare Secondary Payer (MSP)	19	11.9
Excess Ancillary Lines	13	8.1
Covered/Noncovered Days	15	9.4
Invalid MD ID No.	10	6.2
Invalid Total Charges	9	5.6
ICD-9-CM Dx Code	8	5.0
LOA/No Match	7	4.4
FY Split	7	4.4
Other	40	25.0
TOTAL	160	100%

Total billed in this time period = 850

Source: Rejection notification, November 1987.

The flow diagram clearly identified areas where the process can falter and where one activity's output does not match the next activity's requirements."

Massachusetts General's project team was truly multi-departmental, encompassing representatives from the medical staff, patient care services (including admitting), medical records, utilization management, financial services, and management information services. For them, the very exercise of having to sit down together and draw up a process flow diagram for the production of a patient bill was a revelation: It was brought home to them that the production of a "clean bill" is a process that crosses departmental boundaries. At each step along the way, the person involved is both the *customer* of the previous step, receiving exactly the information needed in order to proceed, and the *supplier* to the next step, providing exactly what the next step requires. Of course, the group had been aware of the inter-departmental nature of producing a patient bill, but the discipline of creating the flow diagram, and the explicitness of its display of the process, moved the group from awareness to active insight.

On the basis of the data collected from the examination of rejected bills, the Massachusetts General Hospital team identified three major process flaws and translated them into three goals:

Exhibit 6.5. Medicare Inpatient Billing Process: High-Level Flow Diagram (Massachusetts General Hospital Project).

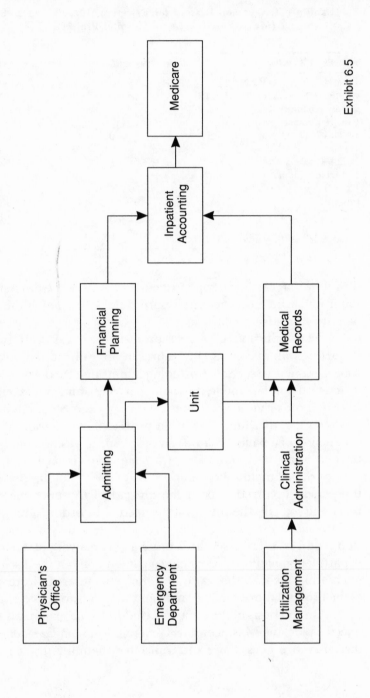

Exhibit 6.5

1. Improve the accuracy of HIC (health insurance claim) number information at admission.
2. Improve the accuracy of MSP (Medicare as secondary payer) information at admission.
3. Eliminate rejections due to "excess ancillary lines" on the claim.

The team then used the process flow diagram in yet another way: to identify the appropriate department to take responsibility for each of these issues. The team had begun with an elephant-sized problem — the high rate of rejected patient bills — and was able to divide it into manageable parts.

Generating and Testing Hypotheses: Two Case Studies

Once a team has used the process flow diagram to understand the existing process, the next step is to generate and test hypotheses about flaws in the process — in the jargon of quality management, "to identify and isolate the root cause" of the problem. The Evanston Hospital and Butterworth Hospital cases provide useful examples of hypothesis generation and testing.

Evanston Hospital.   The team from Evanston Hospital began by attempting to find out what was causing delays in the operating room. They suspected that an increase in the volume of ambulatory surgery was the primary cause of scheduling delays, but the team wanted to conduct a systematic investigation to track down the root cause of the delay *before* proceeding with a cure.

Like the Kaiser-Permanente and Massachusetts General teams, the Evanston group began by examining the process as it was currently configured, creating a process flow diagram to follow the patient's progress from initial contact with the surgeon through preoperative preparation, surgery, discharge, and subsequent follow-up (Exhibit 6.6). The process flow diagram was useful to the Evanston team not only in developing its awareness of an underlying process (as in the Kaiser-Permanente and

Exhibit 6.6. Ambulatory Surgery Patient Flow: A Process Flow Diagram (Evanston Hospital Project).

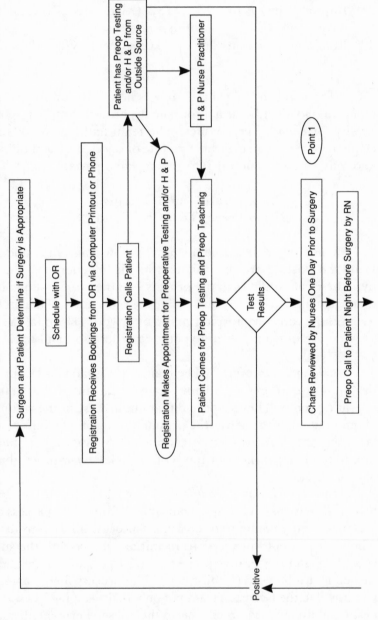

Exhibit 6.6. Ambulatory Surgery Patient Flow: A Process Flow Diagram (Evanston Hospital Project), Cont'd.

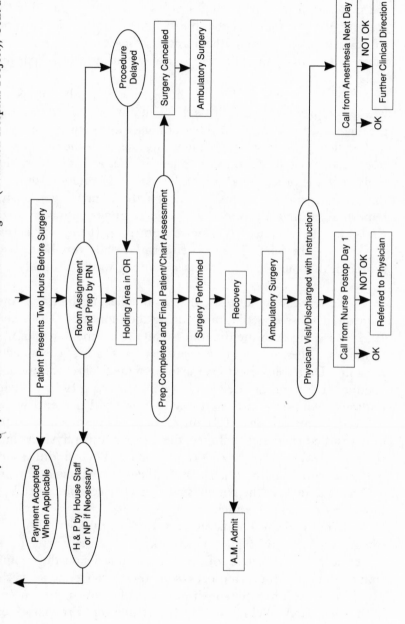

Massachusetts General cases), but *in guiding its development of hypotheses and collection of data*. First, the flow diagram made clear the major steps in a multistep process. The group was able to identify five key points as possible locations of delay. Data were collected for one month on the duration of each key process step; the results proved the *prevalence* of delay but did not reveal its *cause*.

Second, the flow diagram helped the group hypothesize where the process was most likely to malfunction. Examining the diagram, the team decided by consensus to review the process of data flow prior to surgery. They surmised that the preoperative stage was a likely point for stress, in that it was vulnerable to flaws in the process because of the many information sources that converged at that one point. Further, they ingeniously hypothesized that a prime cause of delay might be incomplete charts for the very first cases each morning. If the first cases of the day were delayed while preoperative data were being assembled, then all subsequent cases that day would similarly be delayed.

To test the hypothesis, the team collected data at point 1 on the process flow diagram during the month of December 1987, assessing both the timeliness and the completeness of information necessary to initiate surgery for the first cases each morning. Data collection took the form of medical record audits, conducted at noon on the working day prior to surgery. Their findings: "The data indicated that 16 cases [12 percent] were delayed for an average of 31 minutes. The key items missing that resulted in delay included the history and physical, lab results, and the electrocardiogram (EKG)." Their findings not only confirmed the hypothesis but indicated a course of future action: making sure the patient's records were complete well before surgery was scheduled to begin.

What had the Evanston team learned by the end of the "diagnostic journey" that it had not known at the start? In its search for the root causes of operating room delay, the Evanston team went through a process sometimes referred to as "peeling the onion." They began with the fact of operating room delays, and asked, "Which delays?" The answer: Preoperative.

They asked, "Why?" The answer: Data not in chart. They asked, "Which data?" The answer: History and physical, lab results, electrocardiogram. The next logical question, of course: "Why are those data missing?" With each successive "why," the team came closer and closer to an understanding of exactly at what points, and for what reasons, the process failed to function efficiently or at all. (One Japanese quality improvement expert specifically advises "asking *why* five times" at points like this in the diagnostic journey as a trick for "peeling the onion" of causes.)

It is especially interesting to notice that in Evanston's diagnostic journey the causal hypothesis with which they began when first defining the problem — that delays in the operating room were due to increased *volume* of ambulatory surgery — was replaced, as they accumulated facts and gained knowledge, with documented proof of a faulty *process*. As was noted in Chapter Four, people in organizations often believe that the solution to a problem lies in more staff, or more space, or more money. Evanston's employees could have protested, as have many other hospitals, that the operating room simply could not cope with increasing demand — that more operating suites, or more surgeons, were required to solve the problem. Indeed, the Evanston report stated clearly how strongly they believed at the start that ambulatory surgery volume was the cause of surgical delays.

However, careful investigation of the system as it really functioned indicated that the problem was not one of demand, but a flaw in the flow of work — *a flaw in the process* — that was responsible for significant operating room delays. That process could be improved substantially without either more staff or more money. In fact, adding staff or facilities *would not have solved Evanston's problem;* it would only have patched it over for a time. Until the process problem was addressed and the process redesigned to ensure that a patient's information would be complete before the scheduled surgery, delays would persist. In short, the Evanston group would have been treating the patient for the wrong disease.

Butterworth Hospital.   Like Evanston, Butterworth Hospital chose to tackle the problem of an apparent inability to meet the demand for services — in this case, the services of the respiratory care department. The team began in the usual way: by examining the processes by which respiratory care was ordered in the hospital.

As in the case of Kaiser-Permanente's procedure for ensuring that patients' hospital records become a part of their regular medical files, the exercise of creating the process flow diagram was a revelation. As we saw in Chapter Five, "The team noticed a significant difference between how this process was working and how it was designed to work."

Like other effective teams, the Butterworth group began its diagnostic work by trying to describe the process underlying the problem it chose. Because of the multidepartmental nature of the Butterworth team, however, the members were able to recognize promptly that in fact there was not a single, consistent process for ordering respiratory care services but rather *multiple processes*. In health care, because "processes" often are not consciously designed to begin with, it is not unusual to find that they are inconsistent across units and across time. The team realized that this very multiplicity was a source of flaw.

In order to generate hypotheses about *additional* sources of flaw, the Butterworth team used several techniques to gather information about possible causes of the respiratory care department's inability to meet the demand for its services. Brainstorming within the team resulted in a long list of possible causes of process failure, which the group proceeded to organize in eight major categories of factors in a cause-and-effect diagram (Exhibit 6.7).

To test their hypotheses, the group then conducted a survey of the entire respiratory care department, asking members to respond to the list of the eight major factors identified in the cause-and-effect diagram. The results of the survey were displayed in the form of a *Pareto diagram,* which sorts out and presents variables in order of importance. (For a complete discussion, see Resource B.) In the Pareto diagram, six possible causes inhibiting the provision of therapy stood out as the most frequently mentioned (Exhibit 6.8). Of the six major factors

Exhibit 6.7. Reasons for Missed Respiratory Therapy: A Cause-and-Effect Diagram (Butterworth Hospital Project).

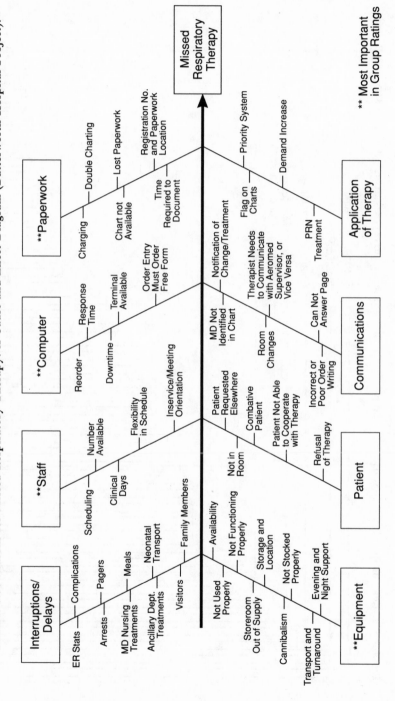

** Most Important
in Group Ratings

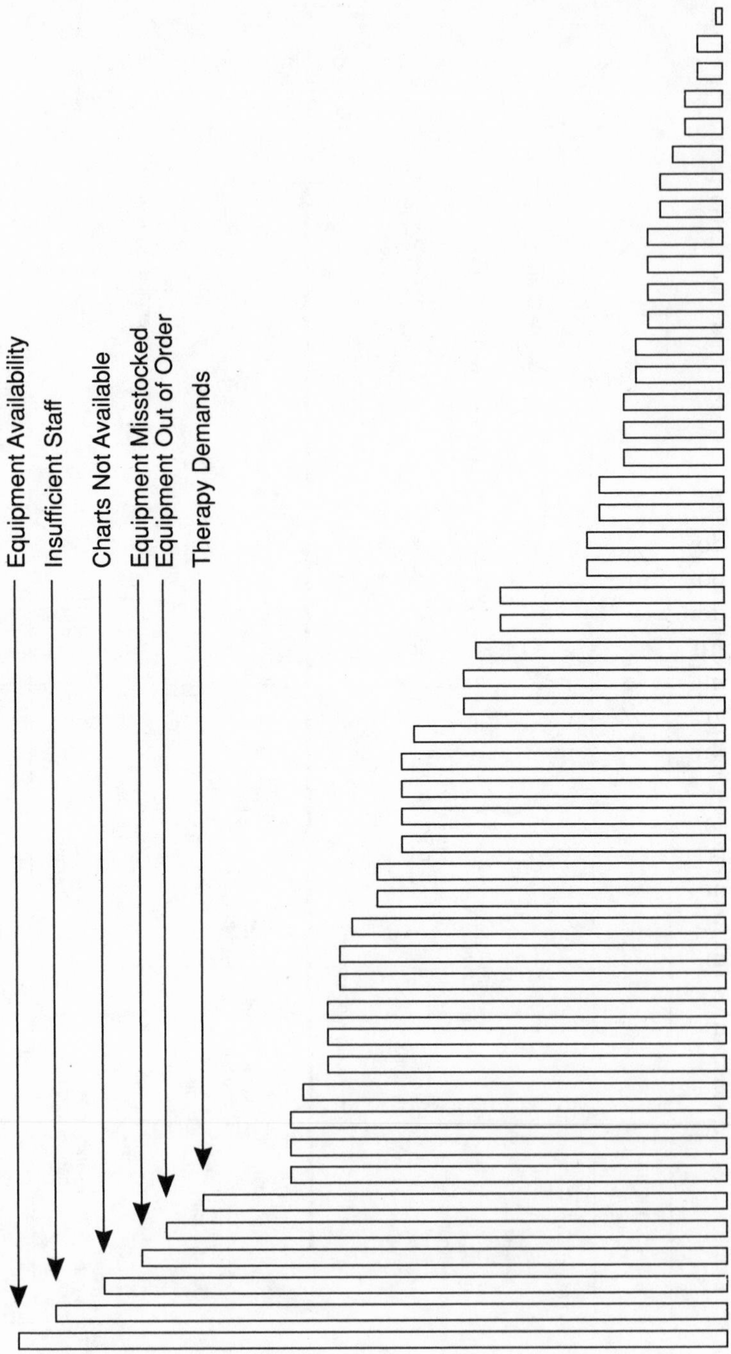

Exhibit 6.8. Reasons for Missed Respiratory Therapy: A Pareto Diagram of Survey Results (Butterworth Hospital Project).

Equipment Availability

Insufficient Staff

Charts Not Available

Equipment Misstocked
Equipment Out of Order

Therapy Demands

in the Pareto diagram, the group noticed that three were related to equipment: "equipment availability," "equipment misstocked," and "equipment out of order." Consequently, the team *localized* its efforts; equipment was chosen as the issue to attack first. One final survey of the respiratory care department identified three specific equipment problems to be corrected: flowmeter unavailability, oxygen analyzer downtime, and oximeter unavailability.

The progress of the Butterworth team through its diagnosis is, like Evanston's, a classic example of "peeling the onion." Initially, the team knew only that the respiratory care department was not meeting the demand. By the end, they had a clear and specific agenda: solving three specific equipment problems. How had they gotten from here to there? They had followed a very useful pattern in the diagnosis of a problem: the alternating use of *divergent* and *convergent* thinking — alternately accumulating as many ideas as possible and then narrowing them down to the "vital few." They began by brainstorming lots of possibilities (divergent thinking) and then arranging them under eight major sources of flaw (convergent thinking); next they surveyed the entire department for priorities (divergent thinking) and then arranged the survey responses in a Pareto diagram that indicated six major factors (convergent thinking), three of which had to do with a single problem: equipment (convergent thinking).

The balanced use of divergent and convergent thinking is a valuable asset in problem solving. Yet, it tends not to come naturally to most people. More commonly, individuals tend to use only one mode — either convergent all of the time ("Let's make a *decision,* for Pete's sake!") or constantly divergent ("Have we really considered *all* of the options?"). Balancing the two modes of thought is a skill to be learned and honed in quality improvement.

Collecting, Displaying, and
Understanding Data: Two Case Studies

In the preceding four cases, we have witnessed groups beginning to discover problems and think about them in a new

way as they embarked on the diagnostic journey. Diagnosis begins with seeing that a process exists; carefully mapping and
remapping it; then using that map to guide the development
of hypotheses as to where the process malfunctions, and why.
These early stages of the journey include sharing ideas and perceptions, generating hypotheses, and generally casting a wide
net in thinking about processes and their possible flaws. As we
have seen, the techniques associated with this stage — creating
process flow diagrams and cause-and-effect diagrams, brainstorming, and surveying — are ways of soliciting and accumulating as many ideas as possible.

The next stage is quite different, both in purpose and technique. As groups move from *hypothesis generation* to *hypothesis testing,* they subject their ideas to rigorous scrutiny. Turning from
reflection to action, from gathering ideas to winnowing them,
they gather information — useful facts about problems and their
causes — in the effort to hunt down the root cause of the problem. They move from the divergent enterprise of generating hypotheses to the convergent one of testing them.

Children's Hospital.   The Children's Hospital project
provides a telling example of the use of data to understand problems and test hypotheses. The Children's team chose a problem in which time was of critical importance to the quality of
care: "As neonatal and pediatric intensive care units developed
in tertiary care pediatric hospitals, it became clear that the time
associated with transporting critically ill infants and children
was an important factor in contributing to the morbidity and
mortality of referred patients." In order to determine exactly
where in the process of transporting children the most severe
delays were occurring, the Children's team started by collecting data. First, they suspected that significant delays were occurring at Children's, *before* the ambulance even left the hospital. In order to test their hypothesis, they designed a time study
measuring "elapsed time" — defined as the difference between the
time a call requesting emergency pediatric transport was received
and the time at which the ambulance was dispatched from Children's Hospital. Data indicated that, "in about 95% of instances,

it took at least 35 minutes for the team to leave Children's Hospital." Their hypothesis was indeed correct.

The actual graphic device the Children's team used was a type of *histogram* — essentially, a bar chart of frequency counts. Studying the data in a histogram, despite its apparent simplicity, can be a powerful way to generate ideas about localizing process variations. For example, if a histogram of waiting times shows two "humps," it is natural to ask why. The data may be telling us that there are *two* separate processes at work, each with its own characteristic waiting time. (For a complete discussion of histograms, see Resource B.)

Next, they wanted to know what proportion of the total delay in transporting children was due to "elapsed time." In order to find out, they did a study comparing "elapsed time" to the total amount of time from the initial call requesting transport to the arrival of the ambulance at the requesting hospital. Results indicated that "elapsed time" was responsible for between 35 and 90 percent of the total time, with a median proportion of 59 percent. *Data collection and analysis localized the problem* for the Children's team: Most of the delay was occurring right at Children's Hospital, before the ambulance pulled away.

The next step was to "peel the onion" and pinpoint where the in-house delay was occurring and why. In order to do so, the team refocused its examination of the data, analyzing the time delays to see if they could discover any correlation between excessive delays and certain work shifts or days of the week. In terms of quality management theory, they were looking for *special causes of variation* — that is, factors that are not intrinsic features of the process but are due to special, identifiable circumstances.

Every process has some degree of variation; in this case, for example, elapsed time might be forty minutes on one day and sixty-three minutes on another. But if, for instance, data analysis showed that every Sunday morning elapsed time was extremely high (technically speaking, usually defined as more than three standard deviations from the statistically expected value), the team would be alerted to a special cause of variation such as a smaller staff or fewer ambulances on Sunday mornings. Their next step would be to remedy that special problem, before going on to address common causes that affect the variation in the process as a whole. It is of critical importance to determine whether variation is due to a special or common cause, because the remedy for each is different. Special cause variation can be controlled by identifying and removing the causes. Common cause variation, being an inherent property of the process itself, can be reduced only by changing the process.

Using the data it had already collected, the group began to search for special causes by looking for correlations between excessive delays and certain work shifts or certain days of the week. The analysis of the data uncovered no such correlations. The group then decided to display the data differently, in a plot of elapsed times in order of occurrence (Exhibit 6.9). That plot showed extremely wide variations in elapsed times, although there did not seem to be a single explanation for the variability. The plot showed clearly that "the median elapsed time was not only too long, but was often out of statistical control." "Out of statistical control" means, by definition, that special causes of variation did exist, or, put otherwise, that *there was no stable transport process at all.*

The Children's team had used data to answer a series of questions: Where was the delay occurring? What proportion of the delay was attributable to "elapsed time"? Were there any special causes of variation in the process? The team was then able to design a strategy for remedy on the basis of the answers to those questions.

Park Nicollet Medical Center.   Park Nicollet Medical Center also chose to work on a problem at the core of which was *time* — patient dissatisfaction with telephone access — and to use data collection and analysis to isolate the root cause of the problem. As was the case in Children's Hospital's investigation of reasons for delay in the transport of critically ill infants, the Park Nicollet team attempted to localize the problem by collecting time data on various points in the process flow diagram. Unlike the Children's Hospital team, the Park Nicollet team was

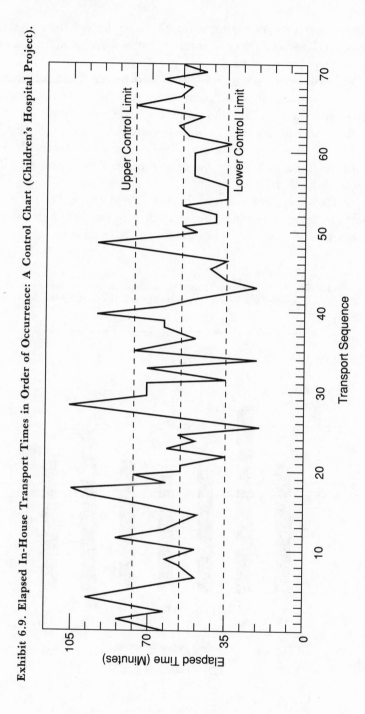

Exhibit 6.9. Elapsed In-House Transport Times in Order of Occurrence: A Control Chart (Children's Hospital Project).

able to make use of existing data: The telephone system already in place tracked data on call volumes, calls abandoned, and average time to answer a call.

Looking for particular times and places when telephone access was especially difficult, the team reformatted existing data into charts tracking "average time to answer" over time. At first, the data were of little use in illuminating the problem: "Initially the charts were developed and displayed for two-week blocks, which resulted in a 'blurring' of a good deal of useful detail." (See Exhibit 6.10.)

However, when the data were displayed differently, to compare "average time to answer" during *one given hour* over a succession of days, the data came to life (Exhibit 6.11).

Exhibit 6.10. Average Time for Receptionists to Answer Telephones (Two-Week Averages) (Park Nicollet Project).

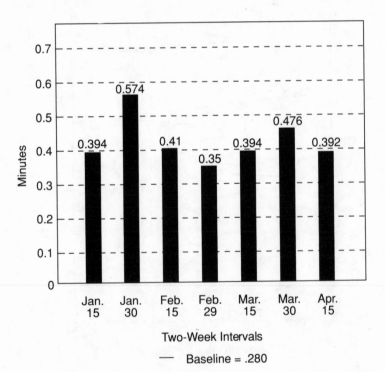

Two-Week Intervals

— Baseline = .280

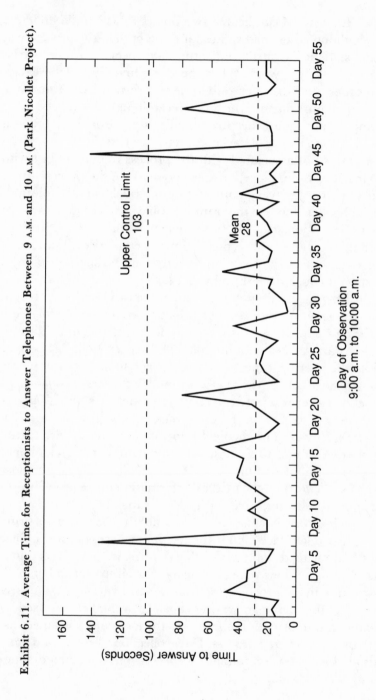

Exhibit 6.11. Average Time for Receptionists to Answer Telephones Between 9 A.M. and 10 A.M. (Park Nicollet Project).

Exhibit 6.11 indicated two points at which the difficulty of telephone access had spikes; at these points, the process was out of statistical control, indicating that special causes of variation were likely at work. When the group investigated these days and times, they discovered that they corresponded *exactly* to the days and hours during which two receptionists were called away to important training meetings. In this case, the data had brought to light a *special cause* of variation in the process — that is, a problem that is not associated with the process in general but with a particular time, place, or reason outside of the process itself. Further, the discovery pointed to a relatively simple solution: Park Nicollet changed the training policy immediately to avoid taking receptionists away from their positions during business hours. The pattern of response times for the medical information (MI) nurses showed high variation but no specific episodes of special cause. (See Exhibit 6.12.)

Having eliminated a special cause of variation in receptionist response times, the team had cleared the way for reexamining the process as it routinely functioned. On reexamining the data, the team found that, over a specific ten-day period, while the average time for the *receptionist* to answer the phone was fifteen seconds, the average time for the *medical information nurse* to answer was between sixty and ninety seconds. *The team had discovered the "capability" of the medical information nurse telephone answering process:* The medical information nurses were taking an average of four to six times as long to answer the telephones as the receptionists. On the basis of these data, the team chose to focus its efforts on the medical information nurse problem — in other words, to improve the process capability.

The Park Nicollet team was able to use data to bring to light two key facts about the telephone access process, facts that had escaped notice until this point: First, that receptionists' training sessions were causing a major, if special and limited, disruption in the process (a special cause of variation); and second, that the phone answering capacity of the process used by the medical information nurses was the locus of a sustained disruption in the overall process. Data collection, display, and analysis enabled the team to make a specific and informed diagnosis of the problem.

Lessons from the Diagnostic Journey

As we have seen, different diagnostic approaches work best for different types of problems. In *all* cases, however, we have observed the usefulness of the process flow diagram. Flow diagrams literally force people to see things in a new way, by arranging an amorphous collection of events into a visible map of interrelated steps. These diagrams emphasize graphically the interdependence of events that may have seemed unrelated and of departments that may have thought they functioned in isolation. One person's or one department's perception of the steps in the process may be very different from the next person's or department's. Having to commit one's understanding of the process to paper enables a group to discover those differing perceptions — often a crucial first step in solving the problem. In the case of the NDP teams, the flow diagrams made apparent, as no amount of explanation could, the nature and importance of the customer-supplier relationships.

We have seen that the process of diagnosis is most powerful when it involves a rhythm of *generating hypotheses* (whether by brainstorming or surveys) — and thereby broadening the scope of inquiry; and then *testing those hypotheses* (whether by surveys or data collection) — and thereby narrowing the scope of inquiry. Through this process, a group "peels the onion," getting closer and closer to understanding precisely where, and why, the process fails.

The collection of data at the stage of diagnosing the problem is a way of testing hypotheses to pinpoint the root cause of the problem. The display of data helps teams *see* what the data mean — to understand the lessons the data hold. Cause-and-effect diagrams are a useful way of picturing the factors contributing to a given problem. For example, Kaiser-Permanente's sixty possible reasons why a patient's emergency room data fail to find a place in the patient's regular file are difficult to draw conclusions from, when presented as a list; however, when the same sixty causes are rearranged into a cause-and-effect diagram, they provide a handy way of visualizing both the major causes of the problem and the specific contributing factors to each of those major causes. For another example, when telephone access

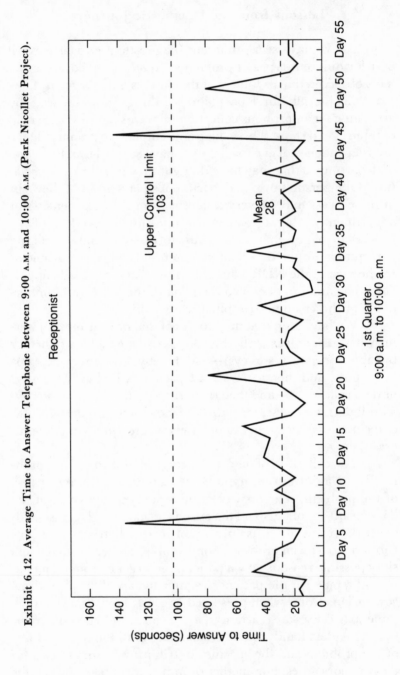

Exhibit 6.12. Average Time to Answer Telephone Between 9:00 A.M. and 10:00 A.M. (Park Nicollet Project).

Exhibit 6.12. Average Time to Answer Telephone Between 9:00 A.M. and 10:00 A.M. (Park Nicollet Project), Cont'd.

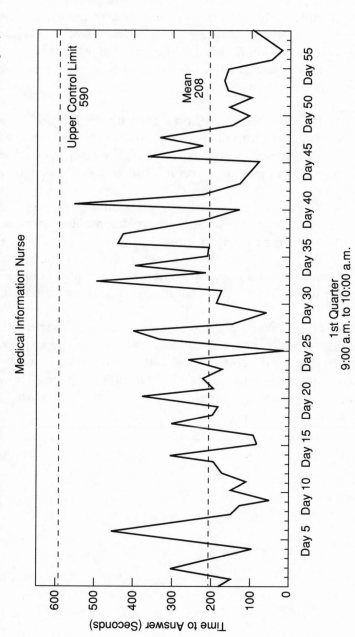

Medical Information Nurse

Upper Control Limit 590

Mean 208

Time to Answer (Seconds)

Day 5 Day 10 Day 15 Day 20 Day 25 Day 30 Day 35 Day 40 Day 45 Day 50 Day 55

1st Quarter
9:00 a.m. to 10:00 a.m.

data were displayed in terms of two-week intervals, they told the Park Nicollet team nothing; when the same data were displayed differently, in terms of hour-long intervals, the lesson almost jumped off the page. *Data suddenly became information.* Perhaps the most impressive theme we see in the diagnostic journey is the element of surprise — as groups come to new understandings of old problems:

- At Kaiser-Permanente: So *that's* why the hospital records aren't getting into the patients' regular files — because when the emergency room gets too busy, the receptionist doesn't have time to get the correct information, or the patient can't give it.
- At Evanston: So *that's* why the operating room gets backed up every day — because the charts for the first surgeries of the day aren't ready in time.
- At Butterworth: So *that's* why we can't seem to meet the demand for respiratory care — not because the demand is too great, but because the equipment isn't readily available.

These "aha!"s are moments of understanding *where* the problem is really occurring and *why.* Further, they supply needed information for the creation and testing of remedies — not throwing more time, money, or staff at an intractable problem, but remedying processes based on a careful and systematic diagnosis of the problem.

7

Implementing Successful Remedies

Once a quality improvement team has made a complete diagnosis of the problem and identified the root causes of flaws in the process, they are ready to begin the "remedial journey." The remedial journey consists of three well-defined steps:

1. Developing the remedy
2. Implementing and testing the remedy
3. Dealing with resistance to change

Developing the Remedy

The first step in developing an effective remedy involves considering a variety of alternative solutions. As was the case at the diagnosis stage, the different perspectives of team members are an especially valuable resource at this stage; since each team member has a unique understanding of the process, each may suggest different solutions.

In choosing among alternative solutions, a team must anticipate and weigh the *costs* associated with each, the length of *time* required to implement each, and the means of *evaluating the effectiveness* of each solution. The quality improvement project team, rather than one department, is best suited to make these decisions.

Implementing and Testing the Remedy

Once the alternatives have been weighed and the remedy selected, the project team makes its recommendations to the appropriate line department. Ideally, any proposed remedy should be given a preliminary evaluation under trial conditions that simulate the real world as closely as possible. This "proof of the remedy" stage is meant to (1) ensure that the remedy solves the problem, (2) ensure that the remedy does not introduce a new problem, and (3) uncover potential resistance to the change that must be addressed before final implementation of the remedy can occur.

Dealing with Resistance to Change

Many organizations discover that the most difficult part of quality improvement is not finding a remedy that actually works, but dealing with resistance to change. While the remedy proposed may appear to be strictly technological or procedural, the consequences of the change may be profoundly sociological. People may feel that they are giving up some of their responsibilities, authority, or prerogatives if the change is implemented. A team can deal with this resistance to change by anticipating its impact, asking "What threats might this change pose to the cultural patterns of this organization?" The team can then develop a plan to deal with resistance by understanding the forces pushing against change ("barriers") and attempting to balance them with the forces pushing for change ("aids").

Keys to the Successful Implementation of Remedies

The single most important rule for introducing change is to *encourage participation* of all concerned. Those likely to be affected by the change should be members of the project team, full participants in both diagnosis and remedy. The health care organizations in the National Demonstration Project that had physicians on their project teams found that they had thereby removed one of the strongest barriers to change.

The second key to the successful implementation of a remedy is to *provide enough time.* The projects chosen by NDP teams were deliberately limited in scope, and this turned out to be crucial to their success. In general, projects risk more by going too fast than by going too slowly.

The third rule is to *keep the projects focused.* The proposed changes should be tied closely to getting results. "Riders" should not be attached.

The fourth rule is to *work closely with the leadership* in the organization. It is extremely important for leadership to be active during the entire quality improvement process, but especially during the implementation of the remedy.

The fifth rule is to always *treat everyone with dignity.* Change is invariably viewed by some as an admission that what they were doing before must have been wrong. One of the strongest lessons of successful quality improvement interventions is that they are intended to fix the system, not fix the blame.

Butterworth Hospital: Simplicity in Remedy

Remedies to major problems are sometimes remarkably simple. The difficulty lies not in constructing a solution to the problem, but in understanding its true causes. As we saw in Chapter Six, the team at Butterworth Hospital began its diagnosis by attempting to discover the reasons why the respiratory care department was unable to meet the demand for its services. The team discovered that the problem was not inadequate staffing but rather relatively simple issues of equipment availability. Their systematic investigation of the problem resulted in a specific list of equipment problems "scheduled for solution": flowmeter unavailability, oxygen analyzer downtime, and oximeter unavailability.

As the team proceeded from diagnosis to remedy, they made yet another discovery. As they looked into the reason for excessive oxygen analyzer downtime, they found that, in an effort to economize, the purchasing department had decided to buy 8.4-volt batteries for the oxygen analyzers instead of the original 9-volt units. Next, the team consulted with the biomedical electronics department, which estimated that the 8.4-volt battery would provide a two- to four-week shorter service life than the 9-volt battery.

The team tested this hypothesis in an experiment and confirmed the biomedical electronics department's estimate. The use of 8.4-volt batteries, while producing only a modest cost saving from the point of view of the purchasing department, was in fact a major cause of oxygen analyzer downtime. That problem had a disarmingly simple solution: The analyzers now use 9-volt batteries. Similarly, the results were easy to measure: Subsequent to the improvement of equipment-related problems, the Butterworth team reported "speedier delivery of service [in the respiratory care department] and increased availability of therapists."

In the Butterworth case, a well-intended cost-cutting move from the point of view of the purchasing department was the cause of far more costly delays from the point of view of the respiratory care department. The quality improvement team was able to look at the bigger picture, one that cut across departmental boundaries, to see what neither department on its own had been able to recognize.

Kaiser-Permanente: Designing a New Process

Remedies are rarely as simple and specific as substituting a 9-volt for an 8.4-volt battery. The Kaiser-Permanente team, whose diagnostic journey was analyzed in Chapter Six, tackled the problem of the unavailability of patients' emergency room records at follow-up appointments. The team wisely resisted the far too frequent, and almost always unnecessary, solutions of more staff, more equipment, or more money: "The obvious solution to this problem would seem to be a computerized central medical record. However, the size and complexity of the Kaiser-Permanente Medical Care Program make it unsuitable for existing computerized medical records systems. Nor did the budget for the project allow us to design and construct a new record system."

Indeed, as the team discovered, the problem did not require a new computer system; what was required was a *new process.* In the course of its diagnosis, the Kaiser-Permanente team had identified several points at which the existing process for transfer of a patient's emergency records was likely to fail. What was needed was a simple and reliable process for (1) identifying the patient's ambulatory care facility, and (2) ensuring the emergency record's delivery there.

The team discovered that Kaiser-Permanente in fact had an existing online computer system that could be used to solve the problem. They found that one of the online systems contained an up-to-date inventory of where each patient had an ambulatory care chart. They then designed an ingenious way to make use of that system: "We decided that within 24 hours of the time of a visit to the Santa Clara emergency department, each patient's computer chart inventory would be accessed to permit identifying patients' ambulatory care charts in SUN [Sunnyvale] and/or MIL [Milpitas]. If an ambulatory care chart should be found in either SUN or MIL or both, then a copy of the emergency visit record would be tagged to go to the medical office(s). 'Tagging' is done by the application of a white sticker tag to a designated copy of the emergency visit record with the initials 'MIL' or 'SUN' or 'SCL' . . . written on the white tag. A copy of the emergency visit record is then transferred to each of the designated locales by routine courier service."

In the new system, the transfer of a patient's emergency record to the appropriate ambulatory care facility no longer depended on the unreliable procedure that had been in effect (see Chapter Six). Simply by accessing the already-existing computer system, the emergency room receptionist was able to identify the patient's ambulatory facility and transfer the emergency record accordingly.

After *planning,* and then *implementing,* the remedy, the Kaiser-Permanente team conducted a *test of the remedy* to measure its effectiveness. The results were impressive: a tenfold increase in the number of copies of emergency visit records arriving daily at both the Milpitas and Sunnyvale medical office buildings. The results of the chart audit to measure for the "timely presence of a copy of the emergency visit data in the Milpitas medical office charts" are displayed in Exhibit 7.1.

Exhibit 7.1. Santa Clara Emergency Room Records
Found in Milpitas Charts (Kaiser-Permanente Project).

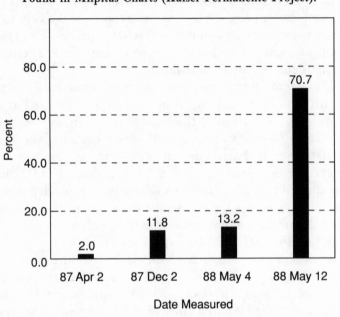

% with ER Records

In the Kaiser-Permanente case, the ingredients for the remedy to the problem already existed. In another scenario, Kaiser-Permanente might well have invested thousands of dollars in a new system for transferring patients' emergency records. The money would have been wasted; the problem did not require an infusion of capital. *It was a process problem, and it required a process solution.* The team took the time to identify carefully the flaws in the existing process and then to consider the existing resources; they realized that the existing online system had precisely the capability needed to solve the problem.

Evanston Hospital: "Peeling the Onion" in Seeking a Remedy

The Evanston Hospital case is a useful example of designing a remedy in a way that solves the ostensible problem without removing the flaw in the process. Just as in Chapter Six we saw teams "peeling the onion" as part of the diagnostic journey, getting closer and closer to the true *cause* of the problem, the Evanston team "peels the onion" in searching for a remedy, getting closer and closer to the true *solution* to the problem.

The Evanston Hospital team — also dealing with the quality problems resulting from incomplete patient records — discovered in its diagnostic journey that ambulatory surgery cases were being delayed because incomplete patient charts were missing key preoperative data. Any first case that did not have the necessary preoperative data available would either be postponed until later that day or canceled altogether, in addition to delaying all subsequent cases on that day. The problem was not insufficient capacity to meet demand, but the process for producing complete patient charts. The remedy, therefore, would require designing, implementing, and testing a new process.

To improve the process, the operating room committee introduced two policy changes: "1. Responsibility for completing the medical record would change from nursing and registration staff to the surgeon. 2. Complete medical records for first cases would be required to be in place by noon the day before."

When the new policies were outlined to the professional staff, they, in turn, requested additional time to establish their own systems for making data available. Once the new system was implemented, the Evanston team studied the effectiveness of the changes. The results were impressive: "Delays of first case surgeries were virtually eliminated — from 16 cases in December, 1987, to 0.67 per month over the three months of February to April."

Moreover, the reduction in delays occurred even despite increased demand. The team was struck by the clear evidence that the problem was one of process, not capacity: "Successful reduction of delays was realized without a reduction in the volume of first cases per month. Indeed, the volume of first cases in February, 1988, was higher than that in December, 1987, yet none were delayed in February. This finding further validated that the process, not the increased volume of cases, had been contributing to the delays."

The success of the Evanston team at changing the process in order to solve the problem is clearly documented. However, upon closer analysis, *the team did not so much design a process free of flaw as design a process into which they built enough time to correct for the flaw*. By requiring the complete medical records for first cases to be in place by noon on the day before surgery, they merely provided enough time to track down missing items — that is, to correct mistakes that were the inevitable result of a flawed process. Doing so certainly proved to be an effective way of preventing delays in first cases, but it did not get at the root causes of incomplete charts. The remedy said, in effect, "Let's do the rework the day before, instead of when everyone is assembled and ready for the surgery to begin." As their study of delays of first cases before (December) and after (February, March, and April) administering the remedy shows (see Exhibit 7.2), the team had successfully eliminated delays. However, there was no improvement in the rate of incomplete charts on the day before surgery.

Second, the Evanston team found that, as is often the case, there was subtle but significant resistance to their first policy change. Shifting responsibility for the complete record from the nurses to the surgeon was intended to "alleviate excessive workloads on the nurse practitioners for locating the missing data items." The team found, however, that even after the system change, records were still being completed by nurse practitioners, even though "the consensus of the team was that surgeons were assuming responsibility for the timeliness and the completeness of pre-operative data." It would appear that while surgeons were "assuming responsibility," nurses were still doing the work. Although the process change had not become fully operational, its intent — to include surgeons in the responsibility for complete records — had been effective, and had contributed, in the opinion of the team, to the demonstrated improvement.

Indeed, the team was fully aware that, despite the virtual elimination of delay, there was ample opportunity for further process improvements: " . . . the frequency with which particular data items were missing from charts remained constant throughout the study. Histories and physicals remained the

Exhibit 7.2. Ambulatory Surgery Delays: First Cases (Evanston Hospital Project).

	Baseline Period	Postintervention Period		
	December	February	March	April
Number of First Cases	132	141	121	116
Number of Delays	16*	0	1	1
Cases Canceled	0	0	3	2
Number of Charts Incomplete at Noon on Previous Day	25	33	29	34
Missing Chart Information				
History and Physical Examination	61%	36%	48%	50%
Preoperative Lab Tests	26%	31%	40%	32%
Preoperative Electrocardiograms	13%	20%	10%	18%

*Average Delay = 31 minutes

number one problem, followed by lab results and the EKG. As was also suggested by the flow diagram, improvement efforts in the future will need to concentrate on collecting information from the history and physical in a more efficient manner." Although they had made substantial progress, the Evanston team still had an agenda for further process improvements.

Park Nicollet Medical Center: Meeting Resistance to Change

As noted, many organizations discover that the most difficult part of quality improvement is dealing with resistance to change. The experience of the team from the Park Nicollet Medical Center is a useful case in point.

As was discussed in Chapter Six, the team from Park Nicollet, attempting to diagnose the problem of poor telephone access, first uncovered a special cause of variation in the process—extreme delays during the times receptionists were called away for training meetings. Next, they discovered that medical information nurses took far longer to answer telephones than did receptionists; the remedy, therefore, focused on redesigning the process by which medical information nurses answered the telephones.

Examining data collected on "average time to answer" for medical information (MI) nurses, displayed hour by hour, the team immediately recognized that the worst problem was between 8:00 and 11:00 A.M. (see Exhibit 7.3).

On the basis of this observation, the team designed an experiment—an hour-by-hour study of telephone access over a period of two weeks—in order to test the remedy. During the test period, they initiated the following changes:

"1. An additional MI nurse was brought in from 8 A.M. to 1 P.M.
2. The 'regular' MI nurse started at 8:00 A.M. rather than 8:30 A.M.
3. Approximately 40% of each physician's daily schedule was kept 'open.'

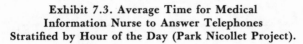

Exhibit 7.3. Average Time for Medical
Information Nurse to Answer Telephones
Stratified by Hour of the Day (Park Nicollet Project).

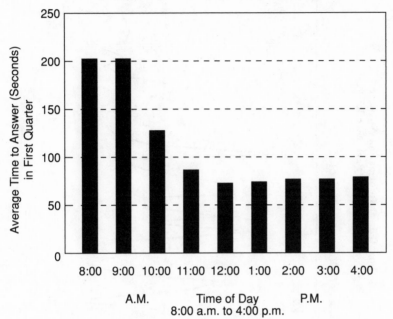

4. Both the MI nurses and the receptionists were
    empowered to use their best judgment to put
    any patient with an acute need into the physi-
    cians' schedules that day, without the need to
    obtain the physician's permission."

The results of the two-week experiment showed marked
improvement. As Exhibit 7.4 illustrates, the average time to
answer for medical information nurses was reduced from 208
to 103 seconds.

However, the experiment had unanticipated repercussions
among the nursing and physician staffs. As the team reports:
"Receptionists and MI nurses were delighted with the ease with
which they could place patients into schedules. Physicians, on
the other hand, observed that many of the patients seen during

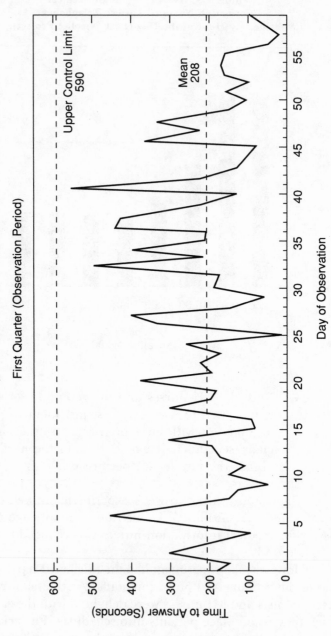

Exhibit 7.4. Average Time for Medical Information Nurse to
Answer Telephone Between 9:00 A.M. and 10:00 A.M. (Park Nicollet Project).

Exhibit 7.4. Average Time for Medical Information Nurse to
Answer Telephone Between 9:00 A.M. and 10:00 A.M. (Park Nicollet Project), Cont'd.

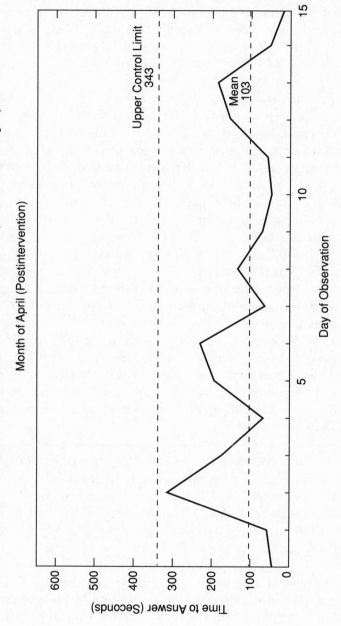

Month of April (Postintervention)

the experiment were patients who did not need a physician's attention and would not have achieved access to their schedules under the 'old' system of appointments. In many cases, these patients had self-limiting conditions which would have gone away before they could have gained access to the physician in the old system."

The process change that the team had implemented was not a simple procedural matter; it inadvertently touched on an important issue of patient access. In changing the accessibility of the physician's daily schedule and empowering MI nurses and receptionists to decide which patients could be put into the schedule, the team was not simply dealing with the issue of telephone access. Certainly, these changes successfully reduced the "average time to answer"; but they did so because they changed the rules of patient access.

Indeed, the change in the telephone answering process made it clear that physicians in effect had been using restricted access to their schedules as an instrument for separating those patients with self-limiting conditions from those who "truly" needed their attention. The solution to the telephone access problem created another problem, at least in the opinion of the physicians; as the team reports, "It did not make sense to have excellent phone and appointment access but to 'waste' an expensive resource like a physician's time." The team later modified procedures further, reducing "open" time to 20 percent of physicians' schedules.

The unstated fact behind this experiment is that there is a correlation between the delay in the answering of telephones by medical information nurses and limited patient access to the physician's schedule. The precise nature of this correlation remains unexplored. As the team concludes: "In retrospect, we believe that we could have made more rapid gains if we had . . . recognized the gap between the family practitioners' ideal practice concept (that is, scheduled appointments, preventive care, etc.) and what their patients appear to want (that is, lots of acute care appointment access)." In attempting to remedy the telephone access problem, the Park Nicollet team in fact came up against a fundamental medical issue: the "gap" between the external customer's (the patient's) expectations and those of a very important internal customer — the doctor.

Massachusetts General Hospital: Variety in Remedy

At the end of its diagnostic journey — analyzing the process by which Medicare bills were produced, generating and then testing hypotheses about the location and nature of process flaws — the team from Massachusetts General Hospital had developed a specific agenda for remedying the problem of rejected Medicare bills:

"1. Improve the accuracy of HIC [health insurance claim] number information at admission.
2. Improve the accuracy of MSP [Medicare as secondary payer] information at admission.
3. Eliminate rejections due to 'excess ancillary lines' on the claim.
4. Reduce hard copy claim errors.
5. Reexamine the attestation and coding functions to reduce delays."

Now that the team understood the root causes of claim rejections and billing delays, they targeted the departments with responsibility for each of these issues scheduled for quality improvement efforts: admitting, medical records, and inpatient accounting.

The admitting department assumed responsibility for improving the process for obtaining the HIC number. In fact, a clearly specified process for obtaining the HIC number already existed: "The admitting coordinator is instructed to make a photocopy of [the patient's Medicare card] for the billing record when the patient is admitted. If no card is available at admission, the billing record is 'red-tagged.' The patient is then visited by an admitting representative, and the family is asked to produce the Medicare card."

The real change was not in the design of a new process, but in a new awareness on the part of the people involved in

the process of the importance of their role in it. The work of
the quality improvement team in the diagnostic stage — specifically the development of a flowchart for the production of a "clean
bill" — had made clear to everyone involved their responsibilities, as suppliers, to the proper functioning of the process. As
the team explains: "Although this process was in place before
the study, the quality improvement project has brought more
importance to the value of HIC number information. Admitting and financial planning have become more aware of how
crucial the photocopy of the Medicare card is to verify the HIC
number information, and compliance with the photocopying requirement when the card is available has improved."

A new awareness of the process *did* result in an improvement in the accuracy of HIC information. The team tracked
the number of rejections for each of three reasons (HIC number, MSP information, and "excess ancillary lines") from November 1987 to April 1988, in order to test whether the remedy was
effective. The results are displayed in Exhibit 7.5.

Although pleased with the overall improvement in number of rejected bills, the Massachusetts General team recognized
that lasting gains would require *redesigning the process itself*: " . . . the
admitting process continues to suffer from task redundancy. In
the current process, the HIC number information is copied
manually first by three separate sections within the admitting
department, then by financial planning, and is finally verified
by inpatient accounting before billing. Through this cumbersome chain, the probability of human error is increased. In the
future, a reorganization of this process may be the only way
to achieve zero defects in this area."

The team's analysis of the current situation and agenda
for the future reflect a new way of thinking about a chronic problem. The team became acutely aware of "waste, rework, and
unnecessary complexity" in the process, and of the need to
eliminate them in order to achieve significant gains.

The Massachusetts General Hospital team next addressed
the problem of "excess ancillary lines." Medicare was rejecting
some electronic tape claims because the claims contained too
many ancillary charge lines, such as charges for drugs, devices,
and additional services. As the team reports, "Such claims (those

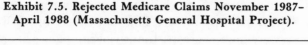

Exhibit 7.5. Rejected Medicare Claims November 1987–
April 1988 (Massachusetts General Hospital Project).

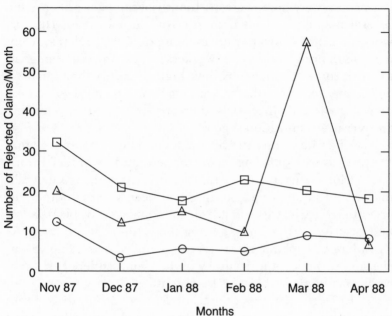

—☐— Rejected Because of Wrong HIC Number

—△— Rejected Because Medicare was Secondary Payer

—○— Rejected Because of Excess Ancillary Charge Lines on the Claim

with several ancillary charge lines) must be billed manually. Previously, our system was not properly flagging such claims to alert our billing department to generate a hard copy claim. Once the problem was identified, the appropriate edit was installed to prevent such electronic tape errors."

The Japanese call this type of fix "foolproofization." The Massachusetts General team inserted an inspection step in the process—a computer edit that automatically flagged a specific error. The computer, in effect, identified which claims were to be done manually. As a result the rejection rate due to excess ancillary lines quickly dropped, from twenty-six rejections in October 1987 to an average of six per month in 1988.

The team faced a more difficult problem in attempting to reduce the hard copy errors. The root causes of the flaws in this process were human errors. Industrial companies have found several major causes of human errors: unawareness (that is, workers do not know they are creating quality problems), competition in priorities (that is, workers have many different goals to meet, some of which may have higher priority than quality), and suboptimization (that is, working to achieve local goals, both quality goals and other goals, does not always lead to achieving an overall organizational goal).

The Massachusetts General team quickly discovered that the process was suffering from competition in workers' priorities: "Prior to this study, the major emphasis in the manual billing area of inpatient accounting had been volume output. In order to reduce a large and growing accounts receivable balance, first priority was given to getting the claims out the door. As a result of this volume emphasis compounded by staffing vacancies and turnover, the accuracy of the claims suffered. Human error was unavoidable and persistent."

In December 1987, the team decided to shift the priority in inpatient accounting clearly from volume to quality. They provided training sessions for all Medicare billers to improve bill-generating techniques. They brought errors to the attention of individual billers. The Massachusetts General team was using an important type of remedy: feedback. It is very difficult for people to improve their performance if they do not get feedback about this performance. By providing special training and feedback on errors to Medicare billers, Massachusetts General stressed the importance of accuracy. The results were impressive: "In time, human errors including miscalculated charges, transposed HIC numbers, and blank fields on the claims were reduced. The result has been a marked decline in the rejection of hard copy claims. MGH received 77 rejections of hard copy claims in November, 1987. This number dropped to 66 in December, 50 in January, 1988, and less than 30 for February, March, and April."

Another of the team's goals in their remedial journey was to reduce the delays in the attestation and coding functions. The issue of timely attestation was important not only for billing but also for ensuring a complete medical record. After reviewing the existing process, the team made a change: "Beginning March 8, 1988, whenever a nonattested record was received in the medical records department, rather than delay the coding process, the coders reviewed the record and coded it as they deemed appropriate before sending it back to the physician. In addition, an autogenerated form was sent to the responsible physician listing all coded diagnoses and procedures for his or her review, correction if necessary, and signature."

The process changes were effective. The number of incomplete records fell from over 3,500 in January 1988 to an average of about 2,200 in July 1989 — a reduction of over 37 percent. These results were " . . . in part a result of a better process coupled with more senior physician level involvement and support." This change made the attestation step easier and helped the hospital gain valuable time in the billing process.

The wide variety of remedial activities in the Massachusetts General case shows just how customized and efficient remedies can be once causes are clearly known. As this team subdivided and localized sources of error in claims, they drew on a wide array of types of intervention, including, for example, changes in process, changes in technology, clarification of customer-supplier relationships, and feedback to individual workers. As they fit remedies to causes, their ideas for intervention became richer and more textured.

The Presbyterian Hospital: Participation and Iteration in Designing a Remedy

A team of administration and radiology service staff members at the Presbyterian Hospital chose to study the appropriateness of the use of portable radiographs — an issue with several quality implications. Portable radiographs are more costly than procedures performed in a centralized radiology facility; they provide lower-quality images and less diagnostic information, and inappropriate use of the procedure may delay access to portable radiography when the need is real.

Based on an initial record review, and using initial criteria supplied by a committee of physicians and administrators at the team's request, the team estimated that 47 percent of portable radiographs were inappropriate.

The remedial journey was conducted in two cycles. First, the team asked the directors of the clinical services to submit a list of criteria that they and their staffs felt would be sound reasons for a physician to order a portable radiograph. The team compiled the criteria from the various lists into a single list and asked the directors to circulate the criteria among their staff.

The team then tested the effectiveness of this simple intervention. After waiting two weeks, they asked the radiology technicians to retain the requisitions for all portable radiographs over the next month. On reviewing these requisitions, the committee found that 28 percent of the portable radiographs were inappropriate.

The team did not stop there. They analyzed the results of their test of the remedy and found that the largest number of radiographs were ordered by personnel from the medical service (47 percent), the surgical service (19 percent), and the neurological service (16 percent). In addition, they discovered that one frequent and clinically sound reason for ordering portable radiographs — namely, that the patient was confused and restrained — had not been included in the original list of proper criteria for a portable examination. They revised the criteria accordingly.

The team then moved into the second cycle of their remedial journey, focusing on the medical service for special attention, since that service had ordered many more portable radiographs than any other. The director of the medical service distributed the list of refined criteria to the medical staff with a request for their special attention to this problem.

After a week, the Presbyterian Hospital team evaluated the practices of the medical service department, using the same process as in the first phase. They now found only 13 percent (seven of fifty-two) of the portable radiographs to be inappropriate, compared with 22 percent (twenty of eighty-nine) of medical service requests judged inappropriate after the first cycle of intervention.

The Presbyterian Hospital team achieved excellent results with one of the most difficult types of interventions—changing a procedure or a protocol. Why were they so successful? "The development of hospital-wide criteria for the ordering of portable radiographs proceeded quite smoothly. The criteria were rapidly agreed upon by various services as well as the radiology service. Directors of services cooperated fully with the subsequent distribution of the criteria to members of their staff. In addition, the criteria were displayed in various locations through the hospital including nursing stations."

The Presbyterian Hospital team observed the single most important rule for introducing change: *encourage participation*. From the very first, they involved the directors of the clinical services and their medical staff. They developed the new criteria for the appropriateness of portable radiographs directly from the input of the people who would use the criteria. They modified and improved the criteria when they found an important criterion missing. They enlisted the help of those affected by the change—especially the clinicians—from the beginning.

University of Michigan Hospitals:
Establishing Ownership of Multifunctional Processes

Sometimes the problems tackled by the NDP teams were complex and involved various departments where people were unclear about their expected roles, responsibilities, and authority. In industry, it is quite common today for companies to accelerate improvement by establishing clear ownership for important multifunctional processes. This is exactly what the University of Michigan Hospitals team did as they set about to improve the inpatient discharge process. They consolidated preadmission review, admitting, concurrent utilization review, and continuing care coordination under one administrative head. In this way, they could work directly on the causes of late inpatient discharges.

The team first improved communications. Within the admitting area, they changed operational definitions and priorities to expedite communication of bed availability. They gave housekeepers pagers and eliminated housekeeping supervisors from the communication chain. They discussed transportation plans with patients before the discharge order was written. They developed a discharge planning protocol in continuing care services to help identify patients with anticipated discharge problems. They also changed a policy so that vacant rooms were cleaned during the night shift, making the rooms ready for admission earlier the following day.

As the team reports, the results of these process changes were dramatic (see Exhibit 7.6). They note that "the most significant impacts have been simultaneous reduction of waiting time and costs. Average waiting times after admission processing have been reduced from an average of 3.1 hours (186 minutes) during July, 1987, through June, 1988, to an average of 21 minutes during October, 1988, through March, 1989. During the same period, July, 1988, through June, 1989, payroll and other costs were reduced over $260,000 per year."

The improved discharge planning at the University of Michigan Hospitals also reduced the average length of stay by

Exhibit 7.6. Waiting Time in Admitting
(University of Michigan Hospitals Project).

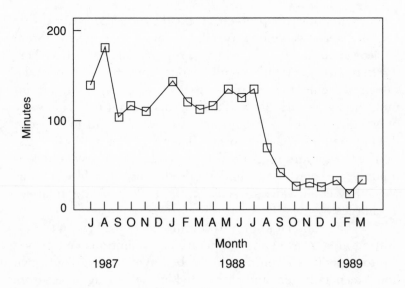

0.61 days for patients needing placement. Since the University of Michigan Hospitals have high occupancy rates, the team estimated that this resulted in an additional net saving of $250,000 per year.

Lessons from the Remedial Journey

In the preceding examples, we have seen teams in the NDP pay special attention to implementing the remedy, testing the effectiveness of the remedy, and dealing with resistance to change.

These successful teams encouraged participation by a large number of people who they believed would be involved in implementing the remedy. They allowed time for discussion and trials and were willing to modify the remedies when they discovered problems. For example, at Evanston Hospital the professional staff requested and received additional time to establish their own systems for making preoperative data available. At Park Nicollet, the physicians felt that the first remedy (keeping 40 percent of each physician's daily schedule open) solved one problem but created another. The team then changed the procedure, keeping only 20 percent of each physician's daily schedule open.

These teams were successful when they kept their projects focused. Often, they continued "peeling the onion" in the remedial journey and focusing on specific parts of the larger problems. In this way, they achieved measurable results one step at a time. We saw the Butterworth Hospital team choose to focus on the equipment issue " . . . because it was the most troublesome and because the problems were primarily contained within the respiratory care department." They further focused their efforts on just three specific equipment problems. At the Presbyterian Hospital, the team carefully tested their remedy. After getting encouraging results in the first phase, they focused the next phase on one department.

We also saw these teams working closely with the leadership of the organization. In the examples cited in this chapter, the teams included top management as active team members. Presidents and chief executive officers, medical directors, clinical department directors, operations vice presidents, and administrative department heads were active team members, not just observers. When organizational changes or policy changes were necessary, the teams did not have to prepare detailed recommendations and thread their way through bureaucratic mazes. The teams could act directly. They discovered flaws in the process, they developed remedies, and they implemented the remedies and measured the results.

In these case studies we also saw a remarkable absence of blaming. The teams treated both their own members and other members of the organization with dignity and respect. They solicited input and opinions from a wide range of people and evaluated the consequences of the proposed and implemented remedies carefully.

Types of Remedies

In the past forty years companies have used a wide variety of remedies in their quest for continuous quality improvement. NDP teams rediscovered many of these. The teams found that many of the processes underlying the problems they had chosen to work on were unplanned. These complex processes had evolved and crossed many departmental boundaries, with no one understanding the entire process. Sometimes what was required was a new process. The Kaiser-Permanente team designed a simple and reliable process that ensured that the emergency department's records were delivered to the patient's ambulatory facility. Sometimes what was required was a simple awareness of the importance of certain steps in the process. The Massachusetts General Hospital team made great strides when they became aware of the importance of having the correct HIC number information.

But in many cases the process needed to be replanned (or perhaps planned for the first time). Massachusetts General Hospital redesigned its attestation process and achieved immediate results. In several cases, the teams established process owners with continuing responsibilities for managing and improving critical processes.

Many teams used another type of remedy: removing sub-optimization. At Butterworth Hospital, the purchasing department now spends a small amount more for each battery so that the hospital can save on total respiratory care costs. Massachusetts General Hospital has replaced the old quantity goals for hard copy claims with new quality goals. This reduces slightly the number of claims sent, but reduces significantly the number of claims rejected.

Many teams discovered appropriate uses of inspection to remove minor problems early, before they could become major problems later. The Evanston Hospital team instituted a review of preoperative medical records for first-case surgery the day before the scheduled operation. This allowed time for the staff to correct any mistakes and complete the records. The Massachusetts General Hospital team implemented an automated edit of the electronic tape claims, which reduced Medicare rejects.

Some teams dealt head on with human errors. Massachusetts General Hospital provided training for the people involved in the billing process and instituted a feedback system so that all errors could be openly reviewed and discussed.

Several teams made changes in protocols or procedures. Although these are often difficult changes to make, the teams made them carefully by obtaining widespread participation and involvement. They made sure people knew why the change was necessary, let people have a voice in how the change would be made, and provided feedback on results.

During their remedial journeys, the teams discovered how cross-functional or cross-departmental the problems under investigation really were. The teams had to develop better communication channels, better understanding, and better measurements among departments. They had to look first at global objectives and then decide what part of the action each department and each individual is responsible for. They also found many more opportunities for improvement.

8

Holding and Extending the Gains

The quality improvement process does not end with implementation of a remedy. The reason is simple: Even after effective improvements have been found, processes tend to regress to their prior levels of performance *unless specific steps are taken to hold the gains.* This decay of performance is a familiar and frustrating experience in most organizations. As one nurse manager put it, "We are experts at fixing problems. In fact, we often fix the same problem fifteen or twenty times a year."

Breakthroughs in results—the real motivation for quality improvement efforts—do not come from short-lived increases in levels of performance; they come from permanent changes: "once and for all" improvements. To make breakthroughs durable, the quality improvement process must include two final steps:

- Checking the performance of the new process (does the remedy work to improve the performance of the process?)
- Monitoring the control system (does the process remain at the new level of performance over a period of time?)

The NDP teams, given only eight months between the initial planning meeting and the submission of their final reports, had less to say about holding the gains than about other steps in the quality improvement process. Nonetheless, several teams

134

were able to begin developing procedures for checking on their new processes, and a few began to follow through on routine process control.

Checking the Performance of the New Process

As a team proceeds in its work to improve a faulty process (the remedial journey), process changes have an experimental flavor. The team develops hypotheses about causes of flaws in the process, invents plausible remedies, and tests those remedies to determine their effectiveness. The experiment benefits from the enthusiasm and careful planning of the team, and it has about it the aura of novelty.

Unfortunately, what works in an experimental mode may not work as well in the real world, over the long term. The quality improvement team must demonstrate that the process indeed achieves a new level of performance in the setting of day-to-day organizational life. Otherwise, its efforts will have little long-term effect.

For example, the Worcester Memorial Hospital team, attempting to improve several key processes in the emergency department, checked carefully on the changes they made in an attempt to improve laboratory response times. Having installed an intercom system connecting the emergency department and the phlebotomy station, and having made several procedural changes in the drawing and transport of blood specimens, the team monitored average laboratory response times. The measurements showed a decrease in average laboratory response time immediately following the process changes; moreover, in the year following its final NDP report, response time remained at the new level of performance. The measurement proved that the experimental procedural changes continued to have a favorable impact after the changes had become routinized.

Monitoring the Control System

In attempting to hold the gains, the organization is moving from the *quality improvement process* (the main topic of this book) to the *quality control process*. Whereas quality improvement is an effort to bring processes to new levels of capability, quality control is the effort to keep processes stable and predictable at their improved levels of performance. The function of quality control is to offer early warning signals that a process is beginning to "drift," and to flag special causes of unpredicted variation that may require intervention.

Quality improvement can be the job of a special team, as we have seen. Quality control, on the other hand, is ideally the ongoing responsibility of the department in which the process takes place, or at least of a designated "process owner" who can act as the organization's eyes and ears on the process. In assigning the quality control function to an ongoing owner, the organization must be sure that five elements are in place; otherwise, effective quality control is impossible. As we saw in Chapter Three, the five elements of quality control are:

1. A clear definition of quality: What is this process intended to accomplish?
2. Clear targets for performance: At what level is this process expected to perform?
3. A way to evaluate actual performance: What measurements characterize the performance of this process?
4. A way to compare actual performance to targets: Are results consistent with expectations?
5. A way to take action on the difference between actual and expected performance: Who can do what when results differ from expectations?

The Challenge of Measurement

As many NDP teams came to realize, measurement is essential in quality control. In fact, quality control requires two types of measurements: (1) measurement of results—the key quality characteristics of the process (for example, in the Kaiser case, timeliness of record transfer), and (2) measurement of process variables—monitoring intermediate steps in the process (for example, in the Kaiser case, proper coding of records in the emergency department, timely pickup of records for transfer to medical office building, and so on). Developing such measurements was a real challenge, as several NDP groups pointed out.

For example, the Butterworth Hospital team, which was trying to improve respiratory care services in the hospital, recognized the need for ongoing measurement but acknowledged that a way to measure its service results was not yet available: "Development of quantitative measures for service quality is needed. Only quantitative analyses can tell us whether specific local actions or interdisciplinary teams are required to achieve improvements. . . . Expertise is needed to develop new measures and data acquisition strategies if available data do not address the concern of interest."

Perhaps the most forceful statement of the need for measurement capabilities came from a team that ultimately chose not to produce a specific improvement project report for the NDP: the group from the Johns Hopkins Hospitals. The team initially intended to improve clinical processes in three different ambulatory surgery units, and therefore initiated a review to "assess quality as a measure of clinical and administrative efficiency." The team began with the assumption that "information concerning these issues would be readily available for evaluation."

Almost immediately, however, the team encountered a roadblock: "Information concerning measures of efficiency was fragmented and anecdotal, with no system for evaluating these data, much less for identifying areas of concern for corrective action. Each location measured different parameters in different fashions, making it impossible to develop an institution-wide analysis of how the [ambulatory surgery] program was functioning."

Not surprisingly, the Johns Hopkins team discovered that the processes of clinical care and patient service were as variable as were the measures of performance. Without a better-defined measurement system, they determined, it would be difficult either to monitor performance or to understand how to improve it.

The Johns Hopkins group decided to work in a different way from most of the other NDP participants. Rather than tackling a specific quality improvement project, they elected to study and redesign their procedures for quality control (or, as they put it in the conventional language of health care, "quality assurance"): "The proposed quality assurance system differed from the existing system in three major areas. The first involved the designation of parameters of efficiency within the system. These included cancellation of cases, major delays, and change of patient status from same-day admission to outpatient or from outpatient to [same-day] admission. The second recommendation was that the system be designated as a prospective evaluation of both clinical and administrative procedures by the staff involved in patient care . . . [to] identify issues as they occur rather than waiting for retrospective review by . . . third parties. The final recommendation entailed establishment of quality assurance groups within each area including representatives from all staff groups. . . . "

This simple description of a new quality assurance plan shows sensitivity to several basic elements of effective quality control. It addresses measurements through which staff can track performance. Those measurements imply a specific definition of quality, since they highlight certain aspects of performance as worth measuring. The tracking and control function is assigned to an operating unit as part of its job, instead of being given to a staff group in a retrospective mode. Finally, the cross-functional nature of the quality assurance group helps make it easier to take action on the findings from measurement. The only missing element for quality control is a statement of targets for performance, which will come at later stages based on understanding the needs of the customers of the ambulatory surgery units and on assessments of the capabilities of the processes being monitored.

The examples from Butterworth Hospital, Johns Hopkins, and many other NDP participants suggest that developing and deploying sound, efficient systems to measure the performance of processes will not be easy in health care organizations that embark on quality improvement and subsequent formal quality control. The teams reported that existing measurements were fragmentary, variable within and across departments, and inconsistent with the definitions of quality that they implied. The Massachusetts General Hospital team, trying to improve the accuracy of hospital bills sent to Medicare, noted: "[There is an] ongoing lack of common measurements or indicators of quality within and between departments. In-house data describing the billing process, including compliance to requirements, are not routinely collected or analyzed. Furthermore, due to delays in rejection notification from Medicare, it remains difficult to provide timely and accurate feedback regarding performance or areas for improvement."

It will be necessary in many organizations, as it was at Johns Hopkins, for managers and teams to pause long enough to ask: What is this process intended to accomplish? How do we measure its results? How do we track its performance upstream from those results? And who is responsible for making, evaluating, and taking action based on those measurements?

Process Ownership

As we have mentioned before, a critical step both in instituting effective remedies and in maintaining quality control is the identification of a "process owner," that is, an individual who is responsible for the ongoing assessment of a process that is important to the organization. The designation of a process owner may be logically indicated by the structure of the organization (for example, the director of admissions usually owns the admissions process), or by the nature of the process itself (for example, the emergency room nursing director may be best situated to oversee the emergency room patient flow process, even though many important people in that process do not report formally to her).

As these examples suggest, process ownership does not necessarily imply direct control over all of the elements of the process. It does, however, imply responsibility and authority to maintain a view of the entire process through the use of relevant information systems, and to convene groups to respond to problems in the process and to propose opportunities for improving it.

A process owner was specifically designated by the Kaiser-Permanente team to oversee the flow of emergency room information from a medical center to outlying medical office buildings. Massachusetts General Hospital went so far as to establish a separate department to maintain and improve medical records: "[The hospital] reorganized the coding function into its own department, called Coding and Analysis, which has set specific standards for coding and which will implement systems of measurement so that the institution can monitor both the effectiveness and the efficiency of this complicated function." It is not necessary to formalize process ownership along the lines chosen by Massachusetts General; indeed, doing so may in some cases add unnecessary complexity. In this case, however, ownership of a critical process was guaranteed.

Reversible and Irreversible Gains: Technical Versus Procedural Change

Although holding the gains is always a salient issue in quality improvement, it is not always equally difficult. As the NDP teams learned, certain types of remedies are less likely than others to decay. One useful distinction is between *technical* and *procedural* (or organizational) remedies. The latter present a far greater challenge than the former in holding the gains, as the experience of several NDP teams shows.

At one extreme, Butterworth Hospital provides an example of technical change. The Butterworth team, trying to improve responsiveness in the respiratory therapy department, discovered that an overenthusiastic purchasing agent had substituted less expensive 8.4-volt batteries in oxygen analyzers for the slightly more expensive, but substantially longer lived, 9-volt batteries that the analyzers were designed to use. The simple remedy in this case—specifically stocking 9-volt batteries—is probably irreversible; that is, once that particular problem is solved, it is unlikely to surface again.

Other technical changes made by NDP teams included a planned pneumatic tube system at the Worcester Memorial Hospital, designed to speed the transport of blood specimens from the emergency department to the laboratory, and an automated computer system for checking Medicare bills for excess ancillary charge lines at the Massachusetts General Hospital. These technical changes, like Butterworth's, are most likely irreversible.

Compare those cases to the procedural changes made by the team from Presbyterian Hospital, which was trying to reduce the frequency of inappropriate use of portable radiographs. The remedy chosen by that team, with the help of clinical service directors and staff, was to create and distribute new criteria for ordering portable X-rays. The complex behavioral changes entailed by the remedy make this procedural change vulnerable to reverses.

The same is true of the changed protocol for handling requests for urgent care visits at the Park Nicollet Medical Center. The suggested new procedure had secondary effects on doctors' schedules and workloads, which in turn led to a whole series of new issues threatening the stability of the initial procedural change.

Other procedural changes in the NDP included the recommendation at Worcester Memorial Hospital that phlebotomists in the emergency room draw blood culture specimens from two different venipuncture sites, instead of waiting fifteen minutes between specimens drawn from a single venipuncture site. Maintaining this change would require, at a minimum, that both current and future phlebotomists be trained to follow this practice, regardless of their prior beliefs and training. It would be no surprise if many phlebotomists who have no knowledge of the original quality improvement project—especially those joining the Worcester Memorial staff in the future—would choose to use the single-site procedure so as to spare patients the pain of an extra venipuncture.

In general, planning and maintaining control systems for changed procedures is both more difficult and more important than for technically based improvements, which are much less likely to regress.

Extending the Gains: Cloning and Spinoffs

The gains achieved through a quality improvement project can echo through an organization in several ways that extend and multiply their value. In the end, the whole quality improvement effort achieves its most powerful results not through the success of any particular project, but rather through the cumulative gains of many projects over time and through the spread of quality improvement methods and attitudes through the daily life of the organization.

Perhaps the simplest and most direct method of distribution is *cloning* — that is, the simple application of the remedy from a completed quality improvement project to similar problems and processes elsewhere in the organization. An improved process in one department — for example, a new system for the transfer of patient records or a new system for timely answering of telephones — will likely have multiple applications throughout the organization. For instance, the Kaiser-Permanente group has built on the success of its initial NDP project in Santa Clara, Sunnyvale, and Milpitas by developing working groups to enhance information transfer between its Martinez Hospital and its affiliated Antioch medical office building, and between the Stockton and Fresno medical offices and outside facilities. In another example of cloning, the NDP team from the University of California at Los Angeles conducted a project to reduce patient "no shows" for outpatient specialty appointments. Having proved the effectiveness of several interventions in the pulmonary, endocrinology, and rheumatology units, where "no show" rates fell by at least one-third, they were prepared to extend similar interventions to other medical specialty areas.

Quality improvement also spreads through *spinoff.* Almost all projects leave a wake of related ideas for other projects. These spinoff ideas are a rich source of future improvement projects. It is important for teams to develop and maintain a recording system for capturing such ideas as they occur, so that they can be incorporated into the organization's regular procedures for project nomination and selection.

The extent of improvement project activity in fully committed organizations can be impressive. Many industrial companies began, like the NDP participants, with modest projects in a few trial sites. With cloning, spinoff projects, and increasingly competent management of procedures for project nomination and selection, today some large companies are reporting several thousand quality improvement projects underway at any one time. For example, the Milliken Corporation — a fabric manufacturer with some 14,000 employees and a winner of the 1989 Malcolm Baldrige National Quality Award — reported that it had nearly 7,000 project teams at work in 1989 and that over 27,000 teams had been formed in the first eight years of the company's quality improvement program.

Health care is still years away from even a single example of such large-scale deployment of quality improvement projects in a single organization. But the potential is evident. By February 1990, one NDP participant — Kaiser-Permanente Medical Care Program of Northern California — had 20 quality improvement projects underway and its medical staff alone had nominated over 300 possible projects for further consideration. Ideas for improvement are everywhere, and extending the gains in health care will depend far less on generating a sound agenda for project work than on creating the means for carrying out that agenda.

9

Ten Key Lessons
for Quality Improvement

In the National Demonstration Project, the long journey into quality improvement began with small steps. When we started the project, we laid bets on the probability of success: of twenty-one projects launched, how many would reach their destinations? We guessed six, perhaps seven. Modern quality management methods take time to prosper; the duration of this demonstration — eight months from beginning to end — was too short for roots to grow. The participants, we thought, would learn methods, but only a few would experience true success.

A few projects did wither before they really began. One participant postponed its project when the chief executive officer announced his departure soon after the initial NDP conference. Another dropped out when linkage to the quality consultant failed due to distance and time constraints. A third became discouraged by the financial demands of the project; though small, these demands pinched in a tight budget year, and the project did not survive. One project ended when the problem it was aimed at simply disappeared without explanation. But the majority of projects continued, and, in the end, at least fifteen of the twenty-one were counted successful. In these early successes lie lessons for those who would go further.

Lesson 1: Quality Improvement
Tools Can Work in Health Care

One by one, these pioneer teams reported back simple, elegant stories of successful application of the basic tools that illuminate processes and reveal causes of variation: process flow diagrams, Ishikawa diagrams, simple checksheets, stratification methods, run charts, scatter plots, and control charts. In the short life span of the NDP, participants formed teams, learned the relevant methods, and applied them. The result was often new insights into old and familiar problems.

In these project reports, we read several times that, through the use of the tools supplied by the quality control experts, "We saw things in a new and different way . . . " Armed by new understandings, the project teams were able to design interventions guided by process knowledge; they were not flying blind anymore. The Strong Memorial Hospital team, for example, wrote: "The systematic approach from the industrial model has provided a useful framework for analysis of the causes of prolonged waiting time, and has led to insights not yielded by previous investigations. The importance of reducing the complexity of the process of care was the most significant finding."

The teams found the project-by-project approach to improvement comfortable. The Butterworth Hospital team wrote: "Focusing on a specific project, rather than attempting broad organization changes, was important. The key benefit of the demonstration project was in identifying changes in our internal management practices, reward system, and use of available information needed to improve performance and quality of service."

Perhaps the most ambitious technical effort of all was that at Worcester Memorial Hospital, which dived headlong into using a highly sophisticated tool — quality function deployment — in unfamiliar terrain: the emergency room. Flying before they learned to walk, the project team nonetheless achieved a clear success. Their experience suggests that health care, far from being hostile to quality improvement, may take to it even more quickly than other industries have. The Worcester team wrote:

"The theories and tools of statistically based total quality control and the framework for using the tools, including involvement of all levels of an organization and cutting across functional departmental lines, were readily accepted and successfully introduced."

We see little in these reports to confirm any fundamental differences between health care and other complex systems of production in its susceptibility to process improvement methods. The health care teams were neither wiser nor less able than teams in other industries. Once taught how, they were able to gather data on processes and then to use those data to make their systems better. The Worcester Memorial Hospital report found, in fact, that "the emphasis on statistical education may be more easily spread in health care organizations than in other industries due to the scientific and technical education that the majority of health care workers have had in their professional training."

Lesson 2: Cross-Functional Teams Are
Valuable in Improving Health Care Processes

Modern quality theory emphasizes the interdependencies that determine how well processes function. Internal customer-supplier relationships set the tone for external ones. Every major theorist in industrial quality control recommends the frequent use of some form of cross-functional team for the analysis and improvement of processes. New teams are useful because formal organizational structures do not often correspond to the anatomy of production processes.

This was, indeed, the case in the hospitals and health maintenance organizations involved in the NDP. When they began to think in terms of process, the participants were naturally led to form teams in which internal customers and suppliers met each other, often for the first time, and developed new understandings of each other's needs. They learned that no single person or functional area has a full view of the processes in which they work. The cross-functional team opens windows that are otherwise shut. Many who attended the summative conference will recall the report from the Kaiser-Permanente group, who, with marvelous good humor, reported on the flaws they discovered in the process of transferring emergency room records from site to site, flaws invisible until cross-functional team meetings began to bring them to light. Viewing the entire process cross-functionally, their initial reaction was to marvel not that the process failed, but that it ever worked at all.

The experience of the Massachusetts General Hospital team, tackling the problem of rejected Medicare claims, also shows the value of a cross-functional team: "One of the most striking insights gained from this project has been an appreciation of the complexity of problems that span multiple departmental areas. . . . Investigation of the root causes of the problem has demonstrated that many areas impact this process. Indeed, what first seemed to be an administrative problem is intricately related to the medical staff and their behavior. Bringing quality into this arena in which no single department has authority or control over the final product has forced Massachusetts General Hospital to understand and adapt to the complexity of the institution's organizational structure."

Cross-functional teams help the organization understand the interdependencies among processes and how multiple, simultaneous changes may be required to achieve the desired improvement. As the group of three hospitals working on discharge processes wrote: "Discharge processes are very complex and require increasingly sophisticated coordination to address the multiple, simultaneous 'critical paths' of communications and actions necessary to reduce inpatient lengths of stay. Simple changes affecting one or two steps in the process may not yield much improvement if other simultaneous 'critical paths' exist."

Lesson 3: Data Useful for Quality Improvement Abound in Health Care

Few of the NDP teams made heavy investments in collecting new data. More often, they applied their new analytic methods to existing data, which they found in abundant supply.

This resource — copious existing data — is an advantage for health care. Many other industries lack similar habits of documentation; they must create such habits from scratch. Doubtless, new data sources will be useful in health care organizations — especially information about key process characteristics — but among the lessons learned here is that often in medical organizations someone has already collected information that quality improvement teams can use. Simple maneuvers like stratification and displaying data over time can harvest new lessons from apparently valueless existing information. The results from Park Nicollet showed one such example; waiting times measurements contained little information when they were reported as two-week averages, but the same measurements gave some important clues about reasons for process variation when the team simply stratified the data by time of day.

Many times, though, the health care organizations needed to modify their data collection procedures and definitions to focus on the problem being addressed. As in other companies, the hospitals and health maintenance organizations found that often their copious, sometimes unusual, databases were not focused on the problems at hand. The old saying that "what gets measured gets managed" only works when the measurements are reviewed, summarized, interpreted, and understood.

Lesson 4: Quality Improvement
Methods Are Fun to Use

In recent years, Dr. W. Edwards Deming has begun to use the expression "Joy in Work" to describe the essence of the culture that values quality. With the transition from the old methods of quality control — standards, inspection, surveillance, blame, and incentives — to the new methods — teams, scientific investigation of processes, experimentation, customer-supplier dialogue, and celebration — quality comes to connote aspiration and even fun. Equipped with the scientific method, the people and teams that engage in the search for useful process knowledge are on a voyage of discovery, and the pleasures of new understanding and continuous improvement are theirs to enjoy.

That is what we witnessed in these demonstration projects. The teams enjoyed themselves. Their reports celebrated not only technically successful projects, but also the sense of enthusiasm and enjoyment among the staff as they explored methods that freed them to make informed changes.

More generally, these projects discovered health care staff ready and willing to learn and try quality improvement methods. Perhaps their receptiveness was grounded in their previous training; most health care professionals, such as pharmacists, nurses, physicians, and laboratory technicians, have studied quantitative methods as part of their professional education. To them, the simple calculations involved in drawing a histogram, a run chart, or a control chart may be familiar and comfortable. They feel at home with statistical process control methods, once they are given the time and permission to pursue them.

Among the happiest of findings was the receptivity of nurses in hospitals to the methods of quality improvement. Many of the project team leaders reported that nurses became champions for these methods faster than most other staff groups. We do not yet know why, but it may involve the "process-mindedness" that is at the core of quality management. To comprehend processes, one must be able to see the interdependencies that all processes contain. The professional training of nurses may help them to see what they and others do in process terms, thus clearing the way for efforts to gather specific information on processes. Perhaps quality improvement efforts, by appealing to the sensibilities and attitudes of the nursing profession, could play a special role in helping to address our nation's severe and growing shortage of nurses.

Lesson 5: Costs of Poor Quality Are High, and Savings Are Within Reach

No single project tried to measure all of the costs of poor quality, but the overall pattern is nonetheless clear: These costs—the costs of waste, rework, excess complexity, and unreliability—are every bit as high in health care as they have been in other industries. In the Kaiser-Permanente clinics during the baseline period of their project, only 13 percent of Santa Clara Medical Center emergency room records ever found their way to the patients' Milpitas primary care site. At Park Nicollet, waiting times to reach a nurse for advice by telephone averaged 208 seconds in the period prior to the improvement project, and 20 percent of all calls were abandoned. At the University of Michigan Hospitals, prior to the work of the quality improvement team, patients being admitted waited an average of 3.1 hours before reaching their hospital bed. At the Massachusetts Respiratory Hospital, costs of agency nurses to fill in for missing nursing staff were well over $20,000 per month.

Costs like these are the hidden toll in today's high health care bill. Taken one at a time, the costs are rarely dramatic. Public attention tends to turn instead to more newsworthy sources of expense, like new technologies or unnecessary surgery. But these costs of poor quality — the penalty paid for routine flaws in routine processes of care — are a major burden on the care system, and they were discovered and remarked on by every single project team that took a close enough look at the processes they tackled.

The quality consultants, who in this demonstration project got an insider's view of the hospitals and health maintenance organizations, spoke with one voice about what they saw: waste, rework, complexity, and variation greater even than they had come to know in more familiar industries. Their estimates of the cost of poor quality grew as they learned more; several estimated that those costs could approach 40 to 50 percent of the health care bill! No one knows how much for sure, of course, but there is no question that the costs are substantial.

A few projects actually counted their savings at the end of the eight-month period. At Massachusetts Respiratory Hospital, agency nursing bills fell by 42 percent, and net nursing salary costs fell by $7,500 per week. At Massachusetts General Hospital, Medicare claim rejections decreased by 52 percent, leading the team to note "how severe can be the cost of rework and how much light can be shed by cross-functional teams on complex processes." Other returns were less easily counted in financial terms. Telephone waiting times went down by half at

Park Nicollet. Average admitting waits fell 89 percent at the University of Michigan Hospitals.

Many quality control experts estimate the returns on investment in the work of industrial quality improvement teams as close to ten-to-one. The success of the NDP teams makes this estimate plausible in health care, too.

Lesson 6: Involving Doctors Is Difficult

Though physicians are party to almost every significant process in health care organizations as both internal customers and suppliers, they are underrepresented on the teams reporting here. Most projects had some doctors on their teams, but between the lines of their reports we read a slightly different story. It was difficult to involve physicians in quality improvement projects. Anecdotal reports allude to the underlying barriers: The physicians tended to be unavailable for work on teams, too busy to join, and, perhaps, too skeptical about their possible helpfulness. This problem was especially grave in institutions where physicians were not salaried employees of the hospital. In such a setting, time spent on a team represented, in the short run, direct income lost to the physicians, who were therefore reluctant to invest the time. However, some of the shining successes were from hospitals where physicians played a leadership role. These experiences show that not only are physicians willing to participate in quality improvement, they can make major contributions when they do so.

The challenge of involving physicians is an issue that has arisen repeatedly in health care quality improvement efforts outside the NDP. Institutions launching quality improvement programs almost always ask: How shall we involve doctors, who do not seem to see themselves as players in processes, whose financial incentives impede participation in project teams and data collection activities, and who do not strongly believe that their interests are tied to the improvement of the health care organizations they work in? In fact, barriers to physician involvement may turn out to be the most important single issue impeding the success of quality improvement in medical care.

How can we get doctors involved? There is room for optimism, since we also know from the work of NDP teams and others that, once involved in teams, physicians enjoy the quality improvement process as much as any participants. The scientific methods at the heart of process improvement are familiar to them. The same methods are the foundation for sound clinical research and evaluation, and, to some extent, they are the methods of good clinical practice itself. In the day-to-day work of the doctor, ideally, patients come with needs, physicians and others collect and interpret data on the pathophysiologic processes, physicians formulate treatment plans, and patients and physicians together monitor and adjust their subsequent activities based on the feedback. This sequence, relabeled, is the general problem-solving sequence followed by any well-trained quality improvement project team. In short, the challenge of involving physicians in quality improvement may lie primarily at the beginning of the effort; once involved, physicians can be quality champions of the first order.

To be successful in getting physicians into the process, however, health care organizations will have to remove several critical barriers. First, they will have to overcome the fear of surveillance and "make-work" that most practitioners have come to associate with quality assurance activities. For doctors in the past decade or more, the word "quality" has meant "trouble." Leaders must confront this fear explicitly and explain clearly what is new about quality improvement methods.

Second, organizations will have to overcome the barriers physicians feel to devoting time to uncompensated work on quality improvement teams, including the time required to be trained. We do not believe that doctors necessarily need to be compensated directly for training and project time, but, if not, they must see how their own interests can be served by participation. They must understand that better processes mean for them less frustration, less risk, and higher productive capacity. They must actually experience the benefits of improved customer-supplier relationships. And they must be helped to understand, if at all possible, why their own futures are connected to the health of the organizations in which care is given. It is the job of leaders — clinical and nonclinical — to explain this.

Third, organizations need to focus on those processes that concern physicians either as suppliers or as key internal customers. Physicians deliver the "moments of truth" that characterize the real output of service organizations; to work most effectively, they must be heard and supported by those organizations.

Lesson 7: Training Needs Arise Early

The time frame of the NDP allowed for only minimal training of teams, and several commented on that gap. The Park Nicollet group explained: "In retrospect, we believe that we could have made more rapid gains if we had spent more time educating the department about the basic tools."

With the taste of quality improvement provided by the NDP, at least eleven of the twenty-one charter members have made some form of institutional commitment to continuing quality improvement as an operating strategy. Their level of commitment varies, but without exception the next issue they raise has been the need for more training. Leaders need training in fundamental concepts, strategic planning, and technical methods; managers need on-site training to guide implementation; teams need "just-in-time" training in basic tools; and local experts (sometimes called "facilitators" or "coaches") need training and pathways for career development to equip them to assist their institutions to change.

Seeking outside help has its perils. The training resources can be difficult to locate, and selecting consultants is tricky. Newcomers can easily be confused by the many proprietary forms of quality improvement education and guidance. The variety of consultants' models may itself introduce waste and rework as health care organizations find themselves lacking a common vocabulary and missing opportunities to learn and experiment together. Doctrine abounds and may divert attention as people worry about which "guru" to follow. To meet the training needs, several organizations have chosen to build their own internal training resources, a costly and difficult undertaking that requires long-term commitment.

One of the innovative solutions to this problem of support has been the creation of local, citywide, or regional networks connecting health care organizations with companies outside health care that have taken quality improvement seriously. In Rochester (New York), Madison (Wisconsin), Minneapolis (Minnesota), Kingsport (Tennessee), San Diego (California), and Seattle (Washington), for example, medical organizations have begun meeting with large companies to discuss health care issues and to transfer quality improvement skills into the health care setting. Recognizing health care as a major supplier to them, these companies often seem delighted at the chance to help in this way; not only are they concerned about patients, but they also believe that more efficient and effective health care will be reflected in their own cost structure. Some companies have opened their own in-house quality training programs to visitors from local health care organizations, a trend we also saw in the NDP, where Ford helped train staff from Butterworth Hospital, Corning showed its program to three hospitals, and Hewlett-Packard shared expertise with Kaiser-Permanente.

Lesson 8: Nonclinical Processes Draw Early Attention

The first projects chosen by NDP teams tended to be on nonclinical processes, such as business systems, information systems, registration and access systems, and systems for deploying staff. This trend was disappointing to some who hoped that quality improvement might tackle clinical issues directly. Some hoped for evidence that patient morbidity could be reduced, appropriateness of care increased, or efficacy of practice improved. Instead, the majority of projects report better business functions of one sort or another.

At least one reason for this focus on nonclinical issues may have been chariness about treading on doctors' turf. "Clinical quality" is regarded as the territory of physicians, who, as mentioned earlier, can be difficult to involve in the activities of quality improvement. The Worcester Memorial Hospital group went so far as to rename their entire effort, calling it not "quality improvement" but rather "systems improvement" to avoid "initial negative reactions from clinicians."

Though business practices were often the object of attention, it takes little imagination to see plausible connections between the NDP projects and improved health status and well-being of patients. The transfer of clinical information, as in the Kaiser-Permanente project, is indeed a business issue, but the same system supports the physician trying to integrate technical care for the patient. Missing information creates a clinical hazard. The reliability and availability of respiratory equipment, as dealt with in the Butterworth Hospital case, is as closely connected to patient safety as it is to capital budgeting. Continuity and quality of patient care improved at Massachusetts Respiratory Hospital as agency nursing requirements fell. And as triage procedures improved at Worcester Memorial Hospital, so, very likely, did timeliness of response to patients in pain.

We have come to believe that many of the distinctions drawn between "business processes" and "clinical processes" in medical organizations are misleading. Pure breeds exist, but many more are mixed cases: Better processes make for smoother business *and* better technical care. The same information flaws that impede correct billing may generate medication errors; the same equipment flaws that require extra inventory may generate hazards for patients; the same complexities that increase costs of processes may add risk to those who depend on the processes; the same ambiguities in customer-supplier relationships that cause waste and rework may frustrate the teamwork that is essential in modern medicine.

Furthermore, it is only a short step from the study of process to the study of the efficacy of medical procedures themselves. In gathering better data on the processes of "production" in health care, we will be generating information on the basis of which we can learn more about what works and what does not work in restoring patient health.

In our opinion, these intersections of processes in health care organizations make it risky to separate quality improvement efforts as some hospitals have done into categories like "service quality" and "quality of care," or "administrative quality issues" and "clinical quality issues." Such divisions may be convenient at first, avoiding conflicts of turf and authority between, say, managers and clinical chiefs, or between traditional quality assurance functions and those of quality improvement, but they may be shortsighted. When health care organizations are functioning at their best, they are single families with missions held in common. If what the physicians want is not what the managers want, then what Deming calls "constancy of purpose" has not been achieved, and a compromise structure will only paper over a potentially fatal cleft in mission. In the NDP, under the pressure of time, several participants moved toward this form of compromise; they may pay a high price later for such structural division in what should be a common goal.

Lesson 9: Health Care Organizations May Need a Broader Definition of Quality

Troubles with labels ("quality improvement" as against "systems improvement," or a "clinical quality committee" as against a "service quality committee") may reveal a significant obstacle to quality improvement in medical organizations— namely, differences in the definition of "quality." The group of three hospitals (University of Michigan, North Carolina Memorial, and Boston's Beth Israel) that worked together on discharge processes put the issue this way: "At all three hospitals some discharge delays were due to lack of agreement on requirements and staff roles related to interfaces, responsibilities, processes, and time frames. The established standards and requirements were not necessarily based upon meeting customer needs. In particular, the broader industrial concept of 'total quality' is more useful to the organization as a whole than the narrower view of quality currently used by hospitals. . . . Many hospitals have a narrow and somewhat naive view of quality, applying the term almost exclusively to hands-on medical care."

Modern quality management is obsessed with understanding the requirements of customers and translating those requirements into internal procedures and measurements. This group of three hospitals discovered that that obsession was not always a shared value in their organizations. Can health care organizations rally around the concept of "helping the customer" with the same forcefulness that has moved manufacturing companies? Do they share that fundamental quality concept?

The Children's Hospital team put it even more bluntly, focusing on the special problems in "customer-mindedness" that may arise in academic medical centers: "The biggest obstacle to systems-wide implementation of these techniques in health care may be ambiguity, especially in academic health care facilities, about the collective definition of 'quality' itself. . . . Cohesive joint clinical and administrative leadership is required if quality improvement proponents are to be successful in health care settings."

Lesson 10: In Health Care, as in Industry, the Fate of Quality Improvement Is First of All in the Hands of Leaders

The "quality transformation" depends on leaders. The first task in quality improvement is clarification of mission, and the second is a commitment to change. Both require leadership. Only the most senior executives can mobilize the resources of time and money that are required for the organization to learn new skills. Only they can strategically change organizational cultures. When physician leadership and organizational leadership are separate, as they are in many hospitals, then the same requirement for commitment applies to both. Neither can act alone with full effect.

The principles and methods of quality improvement, as it happens, seem so logical and motivating that employees at any level, once exposed to them, may begin to use them to some extent even without an organizational plan to do so. The team at Strong Memorial Hospital noticed this, and reported: "We learned that the process [of quality improvement] cannot be fully contained once introduced into the institution. The continuous quality improvement theme has spread to a variable extent through the hospital." But do not confuse this benign "infection" with a full-fledged plan. The breakthroughs in management and results that companies have achieved with quality improvement methods did not "just happen" as a matter of spontaneous spread. The leaders of those companies planned the changes, deployed the methods, and integrated the quality agenda with the overall corporate strategy. Quality improvement can sprout from the middle, but only leaders can help it take root as a companywide organizational strategy.

The Butterworth Hospital team, with both optimism and clarity, summarized their overall experience this way: "The National Demonstration Project provided new perspectives in problem resolution. Surprisingly, most of the keys to improved service were at hand. Improvement had little to do with exotic analytical methods. Improvement required leadership from responsible management and attainable objectives relevant to those directly responsible. The industrial quality strategy of continuous improvement and breakthrough in results provided the needed guidance." But they were also careful to state their specific concern that "any improvements will be isolated and short-term unless they are consistent with the strategic plan and vision for [the hospital]."

In the NDP, the institutions represented at the outset by their chief executive or another top manager achieved the greatest success; those whose senior leaders were absent became the most frustrated. With the chief executive present, the effort to learn about quality improvement and to test it in a project moved more quickly and with fewer artificial boundaries. The correspondence between executive presence and success was not absolute, but the trend was clear. In fact, *every* project report commented on the importance of visible senior management support in the work of quality improvement.

Robert Galvin, chairman of the board of Motorola, Inc., has said of his form of leadership, "It is our privilege to seek perfection." That privilege, and the obligation it implies, starts at the top.

We were honored by the opportunity to work with the many managers, clinicians, and quality experts who came together in the NDP. We began it with hope, and we concluded it with confidence. We expected more than was reasonable, and we observed more than we expected. The efforts of these professionals, dedicated to excellence and asking only the chance to do their best, established a benchmark. We are confident that, with time, resources, and committed leaders, quality improvement methods will flourish in health care as they have in other industries, and that all of us — patients, clinicians, managers, payers, and society at large — will profit.

Afterword:
Reflections on
the Future

by David A. Garvin
Professor of Business Administration
Harvard Business School

The National Demonstration Project was an ambitious, year-long, nationwide experiment. The participants on "both sides" of the project, from industry and from health care, came to the effort eager to find an answer to the question: "Can the principles and techniques of industrial quality control be applied successfully to health care?" As we proceeded, we came to realize that the appropriate question to ask was a substantially more modest one: "*What happens when* health care organizations make their first attempts to apply the principles and techniques of quality control?"

This book has given us a textured and nuanced answer to that question. The cases that compose the NDP provide us with one of the first opportunities available to study the application of industrial quality control to the field of health care. While they do not yet provide a conclusive answer to the NDP's original concern, they *do* make it possible to formulate some fundamental questions that can guide our future discussion and research.

159

To What Extent Does Health Care
Pose Unique Problems for Quality Management?

First, the question of "transferability"—that is, whether or not the principles and techniques of industrial quality control can be applied successfully to health care—depends on the extent to which health care is fundamentally like or fundamentally different from other businesses. That question can be broken into two parts. The first is, "To what extent is health care *as a business* unique?" The second is, "To what extent do issues of the *quality of patient care* raise unique problems?" Certainly, health care organizations share many features with other businesses. However, there are three major features of health care that pose problems—not obstacles, necessarily, but certainly major challenges—to the successful application of quality improvement.

The first, which surfaced in several of the NDP cases, is the often *murky connection in medical care between inputs and outputs.* In health care, unlike industry, it is not always clear exactly what activities are leading to what clinical results. Cause-and-effect relationships are seldom fully defined, especially when the conditions are rare or are seen infrequently. The second unusual feature of health care is how difficult it may be for the customers (patients) to *distinguish high-quality from low-quality care.* Often health status results are perceived only after a very long time lag; in some cases, differences in technical care quality are simply not discernible by other than highly professional judgment. And even highly professional judgments may differ. The third peculiarity of health care is largely an organizational issue. *Large hospitals seem to operate with two distinct lines of authority, the administrative staff and the medical staff,* instead of the single pyramid of authority more common in industry.

These three characteristics are distinguishing features of health care organizations; however, some of them do have parallels in industrial settings. For example, the lack of a clear connection between inputs and outputs is often presented as a problem in managing R&D laboratories. We do not know exactly what kinds of activities lead to what kinds of results, yet we still find that some laboratories perform better than others.

Further, there are product and service industries other than health care where the customer has some difficulty judging the technical quality of work. How, for example, can clients judge the work of lawyers, air travelers the competence of pilots, or automobile owners the skill of garage mechanics (on issues other than service)? Finally, the problem of two lines of authority is not confined to hospitals — it clearly exists in universities, and also in other services organized along collegial lines, where a professional group plays a strong, or dominant, role.

Nevertheless, health care is different from traditional industry in fundamental ways, and these must be taken into consideration when applying the industrial quality control model. It may be, for example, that effective quality management in health care will require unusual self-consciousness and discipline in trying to understand links between care and health status outcome. The attempt to involve customers in judging quality may require an investment in helping patients understand both medical care and their own technical needs. And the dual hierarchies of some hospitals may require special attention to dialogue, conflict resolution, and joint planning among medical and nonmedical leaders.

To What Extent Do Attempts to Improve the Quality of Clinical Care Raise Unique Problems?

Second, in industry, when one talks about "variation," one talks about it from a known and accepted standard. There is a very clear statement of the specification to be met; a part has to be one inch, plus or minus a certain dimension. In medicine there is also variation, such as differences in physicians' choice of diagnostic tests, therapies, or patterns of specialty referral, but it is often variation from a standard that is not widely accepted (and, in some cases, unknown). "Best practice" is often a matter of judgment.

Another problem in the application of quality improvement to clinical care is that, in this area, physician resistance to certain aspects of quality management is likely to be especially high. First, doctors may resist measurement because of its association with policing activities; physicians are suspicious that measurement allegedly for improvement may instead be used for judgment and surveillance. Second, there is substantial resistance to standardization. Many doctors share the belief that medicine is an art; attempts to standardize practice are likely to encounter resistance from those members of the professional elite holding this view. Third, resistance is likely because of an anticipated loss of autonomy. Proceduralizing an approach clearly limits a doctor's freedom to diagnose and prescribe freely. Here again, there are similarities to professional groups in industry; we often find the same resistance among scientists in R&D laboratories, for example.

The quest for "best practices," however, is certainly a researchable matter. It is possible to collect large databases and make rough analyses of better and worse outcomes. We are even likely to be able to develop inferences about what appropriate standards for care might be. We have also seen, in the experiences of several of the NDP groups, that physcians' resistance falls substantially when they are involved from the start in the development of protocols and standards. The larger question, however, still remains unanswered: To what extent does the industrial quality control model need to be modified in order to address the specifics of clinical care? Further discussion and research are clearly required.

Is Industrial Quality Control Truly New and Different?

A third unresolved question is the extent to which industrial quality control differs from the traditional approach to quality control and quality assurance used in health care. Stated bluntly, "Is industrial quality control really all that new and different?" One of the primary distinguishing features of the industrial model of quality control is its regular use of certain tools for understanding processes and for discovering causes of flaws and variation. One such tool is the *process flow diagram;* as we have seen in virtually every NDP project, process flow diagrams served as the starting point for improvement. A second tool is the *cause-and-effect diagram,* a means of organizing hypotheses originally suggested by a Japanese statistician, Kaoru Ishikawa, specifically for use in quality control and improvement. A third tool is the *control chart,* which is a means for studying the variability, stability, and average performance level of a process. It, too, was developed largely for use in quality control. A fourth set of tools includes more *generic methods of organizing and displaying data,* such as histograms, Pareto diagrams, and stem-and-leaf, box, and scatter plots.

The tools of quality control distinguish it from classical health care quality assurance; however, what is truly unique about the field of quality control is not its tools, but its *ethos* — the set of attitudes that it brings to quality problems.

The first is the idea that when it comes to problems, *prevention is preferable to detection.* A key principle of quality control is that the way to solve a problem is to redesign the process that produces the product, or otherwise ensure that the problem never arises in the first place, rather than identifying and fixing defective products after the fact. Inspection at the end of the line is an inefficient way of solving quality problems. Yet traditional health care quality assurance focuses more on the technology of inspection than on the technologies of control and improvement.

The second identifying feature of the industrial quality ethos is *a focus on the system, not the individual.* Industrial quality control holds that, by and large, problems are systemic in character. The way to improve quality is to understand the process that generates problems, rather than try to blame particular individuals. It is seldom the receptionist, the nurse, or the doctor who is causing problems; more often, it is the system within which they operate.

The third distinguishing feature of industrial quality control is its strong acknowledgment of *the centrality of the customer.* Industrial quality control refers to customers in two ways: one, which is quite traditional, involves the external customer — in health care, the patient (or purchaser of care). Another, which is more distinctive to industrial quality control, involves the internal customer — that person at each step in the process who must be provided with something by the previous step (the internal supplier).

A fourth identifying feature of industrial quality control is the acceptance of *variation as endemic*. In the industrial model, variation is acknowledged as a fact of life. The quality control expert uses theoretically grounded statistical methods to distinguish random variation ("general cause") from variation that indicates particular problems not endemic to the process ("special cause"), since each requires its own form of remedy.

Finally, when compared to the traditional model of health care quality assurance, industrial quality control employs *a much broader definition of quality*. It is not simply quality of care that matters, but also quality of service, amenities, reliability — all of the aspects of the health care encounter. While it is important to focus on issues related to the quality of care and health status outcome, it is equally important to acknowledge the existence of a broader conception of quality, because that is the conception guiding customers' expectations.

Together, these five items constitute the major characteristics of industrial quality control — not simply a difference in methods, but in some basic assumptions as well.

Where Do We Go from Here?

Most of the groups in the NDP undertook individual, isolated projects. Having taken those first steps, how can they move from project-by-project successes to an organizationwide quality improvement process? The key is to move from isolated successes to *cultural change*, from activities that are viewed as exceptional and one-time-only, to activities that become part of the fabric of day-to-day work life.

There are a number of preconditions for this transition to occur. The first is *to establish the credibility and value of the industrial quality model*. That is usually achieved by leveraging any successes from the first pilot projects. The second precondition is the need to *educate and train across the entire organization*, in multiple departments, but also at all levels, from senior managers down to front-line employees. The third precondition is the need for *continued senior management leadership*. This is not a need that abates after early successes. Senior management must continue to be visible, involved, and committed throughout the entire process. In fact, modern quality management is nothing less than a new way to lead. The fourth precondition is the need to *integrate quality into the strategic business plan* of an organization, as well as into daily activities.

Does Quality Improvement Address the Basic Problems of Health Care?

One final concern is a profound one, namely, that quality improvement tackles only a very narrow piece of the difficulties facing health care today. As health care struggles to contend with regulation, cost containment, and a variety of other severe pressures, is quality just a flea on the elephant? Might the industrial quality control approach be, at best, secondary or ancillary to the main activities of health care; at worst, irrelevant to its basic needs?

The evidence of the NDP is in many ways to the contrary: the experience of several participants suggests that quality improvement, far from being a diversion, leads directly to greater efficiency and cost reduction. Indeed if, as seems increasingly likely, the basis for competition in health care shifts from a pure price basis to some combination of price, quality of service, and quality of care, then the issue of quality will become fundamental to the survival of many health care organizations. Far from being an interesting, but tangential, activity, there is reason to believe that quality is likely to become an important basis for competing in health care over the next decade.

Resource A:
Participants in the
National Demonstration Project

Health Care Organizations

Beth Israel Hospital

Priscilla Dasse
Assistant Director

Peggy Reiley, R.N., M.S.
Director of Quality Assurance and Development

Brigham & Women's Hospital

David Blumenthal, M.D.
Senior Vice President

Sheridan Kassirer
Vice President for Clinical Services

Glenn Laffel, M.D.
Director, Quality Assurance Planning

H. Richard Nesson, M.D.
President

Butterworth Hospital

Randall Kehr
Department Manager, Respiratory Care

Randall J. Wagner
Vice President, Operations

The Children's Hospital

Robert K. Crone, M.D.
Director, Multidisciplinary ICU

David G. Nathan, M.D.
Chairman, Department of Medicine

The Evanston Hospital

Mark Neaman
President and COO

James Roberts, M.D.
Senior Vice President for Research and Planning
Joint Commission on Accreditation of
Health Care Organizations

Dale Sowders
Assistant to the President

Group Health Cooperative of Puget Sound

Bruce Perry, M.D., M.P.H.
Director, Quality of Care Assessment

Cheryl M. Scott
Regional Vice President/Assistant COO

Harvard Community Health Plan

Stephen Baer, M.D.
Chief, OB/GYN

David Chin, M.D.
President, Health Centers Division

David Cochran, M.D.
Director, Boston Center

Debra Cookson
Project Coordinator, Quality-of-Care Management

Lawrence Gottlieb, M.D.
Director of Clinical Guidelines Program

Diana Parks Forbes, R.N., N.P.
Wellesley OB/GYN

Kay M. Larholt
Statistical Specialist

Johns Hopkins Health System

Theodore M. King, M.D., Ph.D.
Vice President, Medical Affairs

Steven H. Lipstein
Director, Program Development and Marketing

L. Reuven Pasternak, M.D.
Anesthesiology and Critical Care Medicine

Kaiser-Permanente Medical Care Program

Robert Formanek, M.D.
Assistant Director of Quality

Leonard Rubin, M.D.
Director of Quality

Bruce J. Sams, Jr., M.D.
Executive Director

Maine Medical Center

F. Stephen Larned, M.D.
Vice President for Medical Affairs

James M. Thomas, M.D.
Director of Surgical Education

Massachusetts General Hospital

George P. Baker, Jr., M.D.
Associate General Director for Medical Affairs

Elizabeth Bradley
Administrative Fellow

William Kent
Administrative Fellow

John Mahoney
Associate Director of Fiscal Affairs

Ann Prestipino
Director of Patient Services

Massachusetts Respiratory Hospital

John A. Barmack
District Vice President
Hospital Corporation of America

Maureen A. Bisognano
Administrator
Massachusetts Respiratory Hospital

C. David Hardison, Ph.D.
Director of Quality Information and Technology
Hospital Corporation of America

S. Douglas Smith
President
Hospital Corporation of America

The Medical Center
University of California, San Francisco

Mary Jane Allison
Assistant Director

William B. Kerr
Director

The North Carolina Memorial Hospital

Mary A. Beck
Director, Program and Planning Development

Eric B. Munson
Executive Director

Henriette (Hank) Neal
Associate Director of Operations

Park Nicollet Medical Center

James L. Reinertsen, M.D.
President

The Presbyterian Hospital in the City of New York

Patricia A. Chambers
Senior Administrator for Professional Affairs

Una Doddy
Administrative Resident for Medical Affairs

Thomas Q. Morris, M.D.
President & CEO

Gerald Thompson, M.D.
Executive Vice President for Professional Affairs

Rhode Island Group Health Association

Kathleen Malo
Operations Analyst

Richard Rosen, M.D.
Associate Medical Director

Strong Memorial Hospital, University of Rochester Medical Center

Leo P. Brideau
Director of Hospital Operations

Robert J. Panzer, M.D.
Associate Director of Quality Assurance

UCLA School of Medicine

Roberta Killingsworth
Deputy Director of Ambulatory Services

Neil H. Parker, M.D.
Director of Medical Ambulatory Services

University of Michigan Hospitals

Richard J. Coffey, Ph.D.
Director, Management Systems

Deborah Hetland-Guglielmo
Associate Director of Nursing

Ellen J. Marszalek-Gaucher
Senior Associate Director

Mary Decker Staples
Associate Administrator

Worcester Memorial Hospital (since renamed *The Med Center Memorial Hospital*)

Harry G. Dorman, III
Executive Vice President/COO

Laurence E. Kelly
Vice President, Professional Services

Quality Advisers

Professor David Bush
Department of Psychology
Villanova University

Haggai Cohen
Formerly with NASA

Christie E. Cook, Ph.D.
Behavioral Health Services
CIGNA

J. Douglas Ekings
Manager, Customer Satisfaction
Xerox Corporation

Allen C. Endres, Ph.D.
Vice President
Juran Institute, Inc.

Mary Ann Gould
President
Total Quality Management Association

David Groff, Ph.D.
Director of Manager/Management Training
Corning Glass Works

Berton H. Gunter
Statistical Consultant

David H. Gustafson, Ph.D.
Department of Industrial Engineering
University of Wisconsin, Madison

Jeffrey H. Hooper, Ph.D.
Quality Theory and Computing Group
AT&T Bell Laboratories

Robert W. Hungate
Director of Government Affairs
Hewlett-Packard

Robert King
Executive Director
GOAL

Professor Peter Kolesar
Graduate School of Business
Columbia University

Burton S. Liebesman, Ph.D.
District Manager
Bell Communications Research

James Peterson
Manager, Employee Benefits
Florida Power and Light

Paul E. Plsek
President
Paul E. Plsek and Associates

James F. Riley, Jr.
Vice President
Juran Institute, Inc.
(formerly with IBM)

Professor Josef Schmee
Graduate Management Institute
Union College

Debra Shenk
Quality Manager
Hewlett-Packard Corporate Offices

Professor David Sylwester
Department of Statistics
University of Tennessee

Stephen A. Zayac, Ph.D.
Ford Motor Co.

Advisory Committee

Paul B. Batalden, M.D.
Vice President for Medical Care
Hospital Corporation of America

Donald M. Berwick, M.D.
Vice President for Quality-of-Care Measurement
Harvard Community Health Plan

Howard S. Frazier, M.D.
Department of Health Policy and Management
Harvard School of Public Health

David A. Garvin, Ph.D.
Professor of Business Administration
Harvard Business School

A. Blanton Godfrey, Ph.D.
Chairman and CEO
Juran Institute, Inc.

David H. Gustafson, Ph.D.
Chairman, Department of Industrial Engineering
University of Wisconsin, Madison

David Hemenway, Ph.D.
Assistant Professor of Political Economy
Harvard School of Public Health

Marian Knapp
Director, Quality-of-Care Measurement
Harvard Community Health Plan

Ellen J. Marszalek-Gaucher
Senior Associate Director
University of Michigan Hospitals

Lincoln Moses, Ph.D.
Department of Statistics
Stanford University

Frederick Mosteller, Ph.D.
Department of Health Policy and Management
Harvard School of Public Health

R. Heather Palmer, M.B., B.Ch., S.M.
Department of Health Policy and Management
Harvard School of Public Health

Mitchell T. Rabkin, M.D.
President
Beth Israel Hospital

James Roberts, M.D.
Senior Vice President for Research and Planning
Joint Commission on Accreditation of Health Care Organizations

James Schlosser, M.D.
Clinical Director, National Demonstration Project
Harvard Community Health Plan

Debra Shenk
Quality Manager
Hewlett-Packard Corporate Offices

National Demonstration Project Staff

Emily Bliss
Penny Carver
Joanne Healy
Rick Keene
Ruth Manuel
James Schlosser, M.D.

Resource B:
A Primer on
Quality Improvement Tools
by Paul E. Plsek

In their first efforts to apply systematically the theories and techniques of industrial quality control to health care problems, the National Demonstration Project teams used a variety of tools that are commonly used by teams in industry. The experience of the team suggests, first, that although these tools were developed specifically for industrial quality control, they are readily transferable to health care; second, that the tools are easy to learn; and third, that the tools are useful. The last point is the most important. The tools of quality improvement justify themselves — and the effort to learn when, how, and why to use them — *because they facilitate the process of improvement.*

The tools have a variety of uses in the quality improvement process. Certain tools are used primarily *to gather information about processes and possible causes of problems* — process flow diagrams, brainstorming, and cause-effect diagrams. Other tools are used mainly *to gather information* — data collection forms, surveys, and nominal group technique. Yet others are used *to display information and test theories* — Pareto diagrams, histograms, scatterplots, control charts, and other statistical techniques. Finally, there are tools that are used primarily *to monitor and control a process after a remedy has been applied* — certain types of graphs and charts.

While particular tools are most useful at particular steps, the correlation is not exact. One tool — for example, the process flow diagram, the cause-and-effect diagram, or the Pareto diagram — may be useful in several different ways at several stages along the way. The matrix in Exhibit B.1 shows which tools tend to be most useful at which steps in the problem-solving journey.

Two warnings about repetitiveness: First, most of the tools discussed in Resource B have already been introduced in the context of the problem-solving efforts of the NDP teams, as they were actually used. Here we return to each of those major tools to discuss more completely:

- *When:* At what points in the process of quality improvement is this tool used?
- *How:* What is the proper way to use the tool?
- *Why:* What are the benefits of using the tool?

Second, many readers, of course, were quite familiar with many of these tools well before encountering them in this book. Yet, in the new context of quality improvement, these "simple" tools deserve a close second look. A simple histogram can lead to hours of discussion and idea generation if a quality improvement team will take the time to mine it for all of the information it contains. Further, the aim of quality improvement is to "democratize" the use of these tools to *everyone* in the organization. Physicians may find histograms familiar from their schooling; receptionists may not. Quality improvement works best when physicians and receptionists alike understand and use these tools to think about ways of bettering the organization.

Process Flow Diagrams

A process flow diagram is a graphic representation of the sequence of steps in a process. It was the quality improvement tool most frequently used by the teams in the NDP.

Teams in the NDP constructed flow diagrams for health care processes ranging from *admissions* (Worcester Memorial)

STEPS IN PROBLEM SOLVING		QUALITY IMPROVEMENT TOOLS									
		Flow Diagrams	Brainstorming	Cause-Effect Diagrams	Data Collection	Graphs and Charts	Stratification	Pareto Analysis	Histograms	Scatter Diagrams	Control Charts
Defining The Problem	1. List and prioritize problems	○	○		●	○	○	●			
	2. Define project and team	○				○	○				
The Diagnostic Journey	3. Analyze symptoms	●			●	○	○	●	○	○	
	4. Formulate theories of causes	○	●	●			○				
	5. Test theories	●			●	●	●	●	●	●	
	6. Identify root causes	●			●	●	●	●	●	●	
The Remedial Journey	7. Consider alternative solutions	●	●	○			○				
	8. Design solutions and controls	●			●	●	○		○	●	●
	9. Address resistance to change	○	●	○							
	10. Implement solutions and controls	●				○		○	○	○	
Holding The Gains	11. Check performance	○			●	●	●	●	●	○	●
	12. Monitor control system	○			●	●	●		○		●

Legend: ● Primary or frequent application of tool   ○ Secondary, infrequent, or circumstantial   ☐ None or very rare to *discharge* (University of Michigan, North Carolina Memorial, and Beth Israel). They studied *clinical support* activities such as processing samples through a lab (Worcester Memorial) and performing portable X-ray studies (Columbia Presbyterian). They looked at processes involving the *flow of patients* in an emergency department (Strong Memorial) and in an ambulatory surgery unit (Evanston Hospital). They examined *operational support* processes such as making an appointment (UCLA) and billing (Massachusetts General).

Understanding the Existing Process. Teams used flow diagrams most commonly at the start of their efforts, to understand the existing process. Exhibit B.2 shows an example of a high-level flow diagram (that is, one used to illustrate the basic steps and broad flow of a process) of the Medicare inpatient billing process at Massachusetts General Hospital.

The arrows on the diagram indicate the flow of information, while the boxes indicate the various departments or functions involved. For example, the diagram indicates that both the physician's office and the emergency department supply information to admitting, which in turn supplies information to both financial planning and the clinical unit, and so on.

In many processes, one department literally does not know what another department is doing. The flow diagram, or more specifically the group discussion that takes place during the construction of the flow diagram, helps establish the communication and common understanding that are essential for team problem solving and process quality improvement. In addition to helping team members understand each other's departments, the construction of a flow diagram can often help an administrator or supervisor see more clearly the working of his or her department.

Each box on a high-level flow diagram typically represents a department or function that itself involves a complex sequence of tasks and decisions. Detailed flow diagrams are used to describe process activities at this task level. A process flow diagram shows the activities (steps, tasks, operations, and decisions) and the sequences in which they take place. Exhibit B.3 shows

Exhibit B.2. Medicare Inpatient Billing Process:
High-Level Flow Diagram (Massachusetts General Hospital Project).

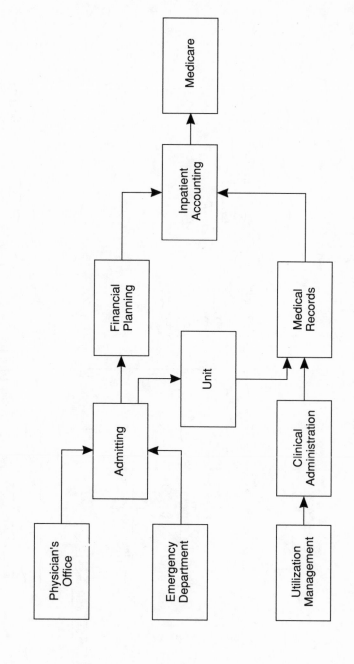

Exhibit B.3. Laboratory Testing Flowchart from Emergency Department Order to Receipt of Specimen in Laboratory (Worcester Memorial Hospital Project).

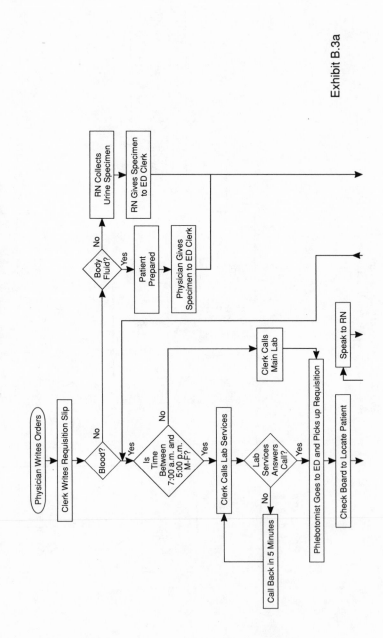

Exhibit B.3a

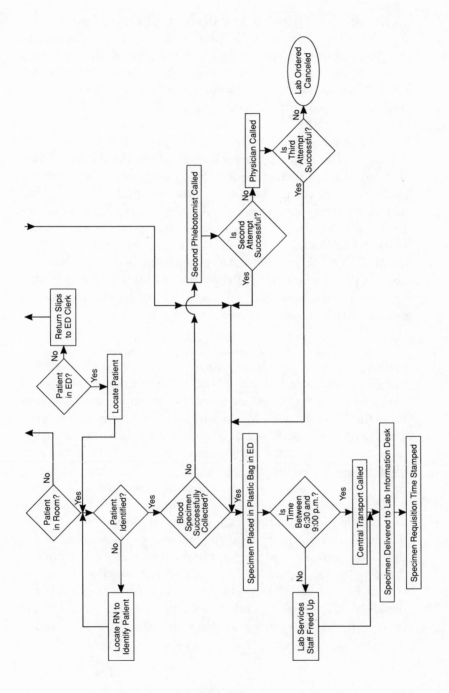

an example of a detailed flow diagram produced by the team
from Worcester Memorial Hospital. It shows what happens from
the point of the physician's order to the receipt of a specimen
in the hospital's lab. By convention, tasks are described in boxes,
while decisions are depicted in diamond-shaped symbols. Arrows
indicate the sequence of events.

Analyzing the Existing Process for Waste and Rework.
A team can also use a detailed flow diagram like the one shown
in Exhibit B.3 to examine the logic of a process and look for
unnecessary or wasteful steps. A particular kind of waste, called
in industry "rework," is especially easy to spot on a well-con-
structed flow diagram. Flow arrows coming out of a diamond-
shaped decision box leading *back* to previous activities often indicate that work may have to be repeated because it was not
done right the first time. Preventing the types of errors that
give rise to these so-called "rework loops" reduces both costs and
delays in the process.

Locating Process Flaws.   Besides developing a common
understanding of the existing process and highlighting waste and
rework, a team can also use a flow diagram to zero in on possible locations of major process flaws. For example, the joint team
from the University of Michigan, North Carolina Memorial,
and Beth Israel used flow diagrams like the one shown in Exhibit B.4 to conduct a critical path analysis of the process of
discharging a patient.

The discharge process is a complicated one, involving
several parallel processes. The flow diagram displays these sep-
rate but simultaneous processes, indicating those points at which
the timeliness of one process depends on the timeliness of an-
ther. For example, the diagram makes clear the importance of
the step, "physician writes discharge order," which serves as the
trigger for the simultaneous steps, "transporter transports patient," "family arrives," and "nurse explains discharge instructions," all of which must take place in order for the patient to
leave the hospital.

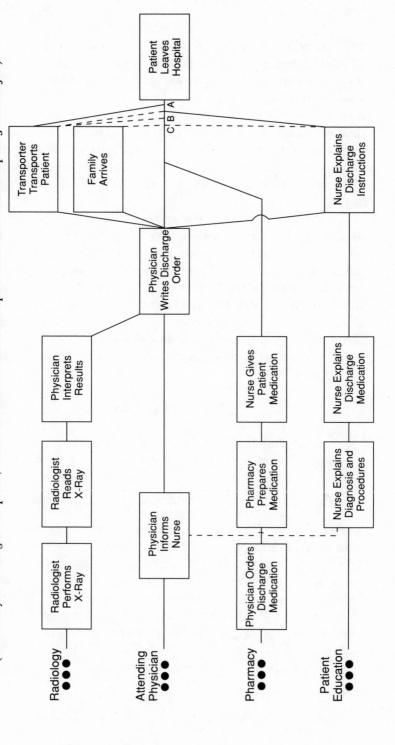

Exhibit B.4. Critical Path Analysis for Hospital Discharge: A Flow Diagram
(University of Michigan Hospitals, North Carolina Memorial Hospital and Beth Israel Hospital Joint Project).

Guiding Hypothesis Generation.   The team from Strong Memorial used a high-level flow diagram of a patient's progress through its emergency department to compare ideal and actual waiting and processing times. They then used the same flow diagram to guide a brainstorming session about the causes of time delays in the system. For each activity on the flow diagram, they asked the question, "What kinds of things go wrong in this activity and cause delays?" The flow diagram gave the team a systematic way to think about the many possible causes of delay.

Representing the New Process.   Flow diagrams were also used by the Harvard Community Health Plan team to communicate a new standard protocol for the management of a clinical indication for ultrasonography (intrauterine growth retardation). Unlike the several teams that used flow diagrams in the early stages of their work to understand the existing process and analyze it for possible sources of flaw, the Harvard Community Health Plan team used a flow diagram as one of the final steps, to specify the new, improved process for making a clinical decision.

Pareto Diagrams

Identifying the "Vital Few."   Pareto diagrams are to quality improvement what triage is to emergency medical care. Both involve surveying the many cases that require treatment and selecting those most urgently in need of attention.

The Pareto diagram is named after the Italian economist Vilfredo Pareto (1848–1923), who observed that relatively few citizens held most of the wealth in an economic system. In the 1950s, quality expert Dr. Joseph M. Juran noted that Pareto's observation held true not just in economics but in a variety of industrial situations as well. Juran formulated the "Pareto principle," which states that *whenever a number of individual factors contribute to some overall effect, relatively few of those items account for the bulk of the effect.*

For example, we might observe that:

- Seventy-eight percent of an industrial manufacturing company's revenues come from its fifteen largest customers.
- The ten most frequently performed procedures in a medical practice account for 81 percent of the practice's revenues.
- Seventy percent of the referrals to a cardiac catheterization laboratory come from only three specific sources.

The Pareto principle also applies to quality problems in processes. For example, we might find that:

- While a manufacturer makes twenty different products, five of those products account for 75 percent of its customer complaints.
- While there are twelve distinct steps in the process of transferring a patient out of an intensive care unit into a standard bed, two of those steps account for 82 percent of the total time in the process.
- While there are twenty-seven items on the admissions forms, 65 percent of the errors occur on only six of the items.

Juran has suggested that the few items that account for the majority of the effect be called the "vital few," as distinguished from the numerous other factors that also operate (the "useful many"). In practice, it is critically important to identify these "vital few" quality problems. A quality improvement team need not solve every problem, or address every issue, in order to make noticeable improvements. Focusing on the vital few enables a quality improvement team to achieve the highest return on the investment of its resources and effort.

Pareto analysis is a two-step process designed to identify the vital few: first, *gathering data* on contributing factors, and second, *displaying the data* in a meaningful way. Pareto diagrams are a type of bar chart in which the various factors that contribute to some overall effect are arranged in order from the largest to the smallest (in order of frequency). This ordering of the categories highlights the vital few.

Pareto analysis is useful at several points in the quality

improvement process. The Harvard Community Health Plan team used Pareto analysis at the start—to help define the problem. One of the goals of this project team was to develop clinical guidelines for the use of ultrasound testing. Their hope was that formal guidelines would reduce variation in the ordering of tests, thereby improving the quality of the process and thus, it was hoped, the quality of care.

The team used Pareto analysis to help them identify the vital few reasons why physicians were currently ordering ultrasound tests for pregnant women. The team collected data on physicians' indications for ordering ultrasounds over a three-month period and displayed the data in the Pareto diagram in Exhibit B.5.

The diagram shows the reasons for ordering ultrasounds arranged in a bar chart in order of most to least frequently mentioned. While a total of 741 ultrasound tests were performed (the total of all of the bars), the top *two* categories—"dating" and "small for gestational age"—accounted for 47 percent of the tests ([193 + 152]/741). Pareto analysis had helped the team identify the "vital few"; these would be the indications for which the team would first consider developing clinical guidelines.

The team from the Park Nicollet Medical Center also used Pareto analysis to help define and focus the problem. The family practice unit of the center had conducted a patient satisfaction survey and identified seventeen categories in which patients had given the practice a "poor" or "fair" rating. In other words, there were potentially seventeen problems to address in order to improve patient satisfaction.

Using Pareto analysis to help focus the problem, the team displayed the data in the form of a Pareto diagram, arranging categories in order of frequency of mention (see Exhibit B.6).

As the Pareto diagram in Exhibit B.6 clearly shows, four categories—ability to get through on phone, communication about new services, ease of getting appointment, and waiting time in reception area—accounted for 55 percent of the poor/fair ratings. Again, the tool had helped identify the "vital few." Instead of setting to work on *seventeen* different problems, the team found that a significant reduction in the number of negative

Exhibit B.5. Reasons for Ultrasound: A Pareto Diagram (Harvard Community Health Plan Project).

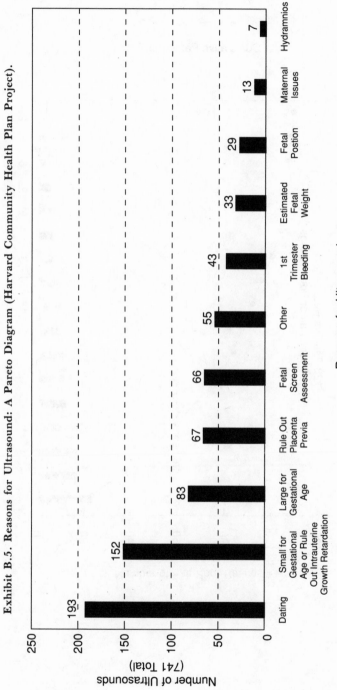

Exhibit B.6. Reasons for Patient Dissatisfaction: A Pareto Diagram (Park Nicollet Project).

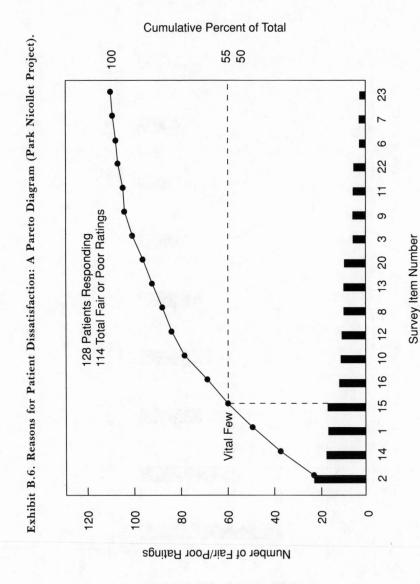

Exhibit B.6. Reasons for Patient Dissatisfaction: A Pareto Diagram (Park Nicollet Project), Cont'd.

1. Ease of getting appointment
2. Ability to get through on phone
3. Attitude of phone receptionist
4. Attitude of clinic receptionist
5. Attitude of nurses
6. Willingness of staff to answer questions
7. Cleanliness of clinic
8. Ease of getting around in clinic
9. Attitude of lab personnel
10. Timely response to phone calls
11. Timely prescription refills
12. Billing process

13. Response to complaints
14. Communication about new services
15. Waiting time in reception area
16. Waiting time in examination room
17. Friendliness of doctor
18. Competence of doctor
19. Responsiveness of doctor
20. Amount of time spent with doctor
21. Concern shown by doctor
22. Information given you about diagnosis
23. Overall satisfaction

ratings could be achieved by focusing their efforts on only *four* problems.

Note that Park Nicollet's Pareto diagram is a combination of a bar chart and a line graph, with the line graph showing the cumulative percent of total for the categories. This line graph indicates that the first four categories account for 55 percent of the total, the first seven categories account for about 75 percent, and so on. This form of the Pareto diagram illustrates the Pareto principle more clearly than the simple ordered bar chart of Exhibit B.5 (although, in practice, both formats are widely used).

Cause-and-Effect Diagrams

The cause-and-effect diagram is a tool for capturing, displaying, and classifying the various theories about the causes of a problem. (The diagram was first introduced by Dr. Kaoru Ishikawa in Japan in the 1950s, and is sometimes referred to as the Ishikawa diagram.) Team members often question the need for such discussion of possible causes. "After all," they think, "*everyone* knows what causes this problem." But when teams assemble, they typically discover that "everyone knows" something different. In fact, there are often as many different theories about causes as there are people on the team. Because everyone sees the problem from an individual vantage point, they may have very different ideas about what causes it. Combining these differing perceptions is a useful step in improving quality. It increases "process knowledge."

Exhibit B.7 shows an example of a cause-and-effect diagram from the report by the team from Kaiser-Permanente.

The issue of interest to the team was the "timely transfer of hospital emergency room data to satellite medical office buildings." This "effect" is shown in the box at the right of the diagram. When the team met to discuss the causes for delays in the transfer of this important data, some twenty-four theories were advanced. The group recognized, however, that many of the theories were interrelated; several contributing factors could be subsumed under major factors.

The cause-and-effect diagram is a graphic display of these

Exhibit B.7. Producing Timely Transfer of Emergency Room Records:
A Cause-and-Effect Diagram (Kaiser-Permanente Project).

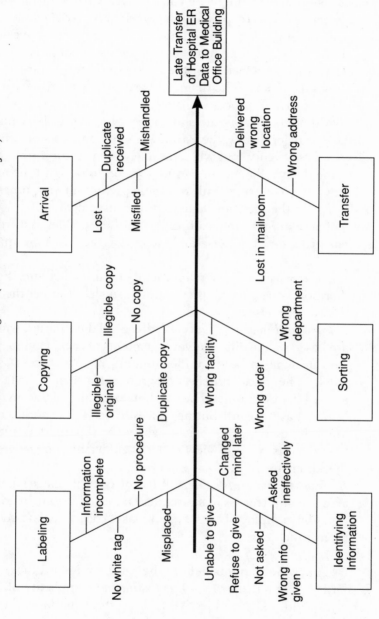

relationships. For example, Exhibit B.7 shows that delays in the transfer of data might be caused by a variety of foul-ups in the *copying process* (copy illegible, original record illegible, no copy made, or duplicate copies made). Alternatively, the cause of the problem might be in the *sorting process* (records might be sorted to the wrong facility or the wrong department, or sorted in the wrong order). The diagram is read in a similar fashion for each of the subprocesses listed.

Although the diagram shows twenty-four possible causes for data-transfer delays, the Pareto principle suggests that only a few of these twenty-four will most likely account for the majority of the delays. The team can now go on to design tests and collect data to confirm or rule out these preliminary hypotheses and identify the vital few causes of process flaw.

There are a number of important benefits derived from the construction of a cause-and-effect diagram in a group:

- *It aids teamwork.* Every team member can contribute. Furthermore, one person's theory might suggest another theory to someone else.
- *It deepens understanding.* The collection of all the theories, which are based on the different vantage points of each team member, provides a better understanding of the process as a whole. The cause-and-effect diagram can also help the team avoid bias or "tunnel vision." For example, if one major branch has ten contributing causes listed while another has only one or two, the team might want to consider if it is biased in its point of view or lacks sufficient knowledge in the latter area.
- *It identifies data needs.* The full list of possible causes helps assure completeness in subsequent data collection. In addition, the grouping of causes often makes collecting data about them much easier.

The overarching benefit of the cause-and-effect diagram is that it forces a team to stop, consider the complexity of the problem, and take an objective look at all of the factors that might cause it. Just as the process flow diagram gives a team a structured and disciplined way to understand the existing process, the cause-and-effect diagram provides a structured way to generate hypotheses about sources of process flaw. Without the mind-opening discipline imposed by the cause-and-effect diagram, teams seem to naturally latch on to one or two hypotheses and begin pursuing solutions without first confirming their hypotheses. While these one or two causes might well be the ones associated with the most recent occurrence of the problem, or some vividly remembered past occurrence, they may not be the true causes in the majority of cases. In other words, eliminating these one or two may not significantly reduce the frequency of future occurrences of the problem. Unless the team takes the time to think about all the possible causes, the most important causes of the chronic problem may go undiagnosed.

Grouping of Causes: The "5 Ms" and the "5 Ps"

The cause-and-effect diagram shown in Exhibit B.7 shows the causes grouped by subprocess or major activity in the process flow. Such a grouping is often a natural outgrowth of an earlier process flow diagram. Another common grouping of the causes is by generic elements of the system. In manufacturing applications, these generic elements are called the "5 Ms": man, machines, materials, methods, and measurements. Nonmanufacturing systems consist of similar generic elements, sometimes called the "5 Ps": patrons (those who use the system), people (those who work in the system), provisions (supplies), places (the work environment), and procedures (the methods and rules of work).

To construct a cause-and-effect diagram using the "5 Ps," the team assembles and organizes its brainstorming around the following questions:

- What patrons, people, provisions, places, and procedures are used in this process?
- How might these patrons, people, provisions, places, and procedures be the cause of the problem we are studying?

In response to the second question, the team might theorize that the problem exists because the *patrons* do not give the correct information, the *people* are not properly trained, the *provisions* are defective, the *place* is physically disorganized, or the *procedures* are incomplete or cumbersome. Each theory is shown on the diagram under one of the "5 P" headings. Of course, depending on the problem they have chosen, the team might substitute more specific headings for each of the five Ps. For example, "patrons" might be replaced by two headings, one for "in-patients" and another for "out-patients." "Nurses" or "doctors" might be used in place of the generic "people." One word of caution: Organizing around the "5 Ps" or the "5 Ms" is meant to help *generate* hypotheses; it should never *prevent* identifying other plausible categories.

A quality improvement team can usually construct a cause-and-effect diagram listing twenty to thirty possible causes in about half an hour. This minor investment of time can prevent hours of wasted effort and frustration in subsequent data collection and analysis.

Opinion-Based Tools

A number of tools have been introduced over the years to help industrial quality improvement teams solicit and utilize the opinions, perceptions, and judgment of others in the work process. Four such techniques — Delphi studies, the nominal group process, affinity diagrams, and interrelationship diagraphs — were employed by teams in the NDP.

The formal Delphi technique asks individuals anonymously to estimate unknown quantities or to create lists of ideas, combines the estimates or lists, and then (still preserving anonymity) feeds the group's results back again to the individuals for reestimation. This iterative, anonymous group process can be used over and over again until the surveyor is satisfied with the degree of convergence obtained.

The three-hospital joint group from the University of Michigan, North Carolina Memorial, and Beth Israel Hospitals used the Delphi technique to study the possible causes for discharge delays. In all, 41 different perceived reasons for delays in discharge were identified from a total of 137 respondents. These were then rank-ordered in a second Delphi survey.

The Harvard Community Health Plan team used the nominal group process to collect expert opinions during the development of guidelines for ultrasound testing. The nominal group method, like Delphi, allows individuals to contribute their ideas without critical comments from others, but it does permit discussion (and loss of anonymity) in group meetings as members seek clarification of each other's ideas. The nominal group process at the Harvard Community Health Plan helped build consensus among clinicians around the new guidelines for ultrasound use.

The team from Worcester Memorial Hospital used two relatively new quality management tools — affinity diagrams and interrelationship diagraphs — to identify and organize customer expectations for emergency services. To construct an affinity diagram, team members write their individual ideas about the issue under discussion (in this case, customer expectations for emergency services) on cards. These cards are randomly spread out on a table. Team members then collect groups of cards that express related ideas. The resulting display of these groups of related ideas is called an affinity diagram.

An interrelationship diagraph can be used to display this same information, with the addition of lines and arrows to show the logical or time-sequence connections between the individual ideas. Both tools help build consensus among team members about the relationships among their individual ideas and opinions.

Consensus-Building Tools: A Caution

Nominal group, Delphi, and other group process methods can help to collect and sort ideas, but they do not *create* new information. While such consensus-building processes are very useful for involving everyone and gathering their perceptions and opinions, a quality improvement team must remember to verify the results with hard facts from the process before making a major investment in changes. For example, the Delphi study about patient discharge delays at North Carolina Memorial Hospital identified "patient's family unaware of need for discharge" as the top cause for the discharge delays, *as perceived by the doctors and nurses in the survey.* However, follow-up chart reviews and a telephone survey of recently discharged patients failed to identify even a single case of discharge delay caused by poor communication with the patient's family. In sound quality improvement efforts, group process methods for generating hypotheses must be balanced by real data to test those hypotheses.

Data-Collection Forms

The collection of data is fundamental to quality improvement. A quality improvement team that would begin implementing solutions without first gathering data to determine the true extent and cause of a problem is like the doctor who would recommend a complex treatment after only cursory examination of a patient. The collection and analysis of data is quality management's version of a complete battery of medical diagnostic tests.

The barrier that many quality teams encounter is that the data they need simply do not exist. Indeed, the absence of data is the major reason why so many problems go unsolved for so long. In order to get the facts to solve the problem, the team must first collect its own data.

Unfortunately, to many people the term "data collection" implies elaborate, computer-based systems or precise measurement instruments. The thought of the cost and effort required to set up such a system is enough to drive even the most dedicated quality improvement team to take the default approach — gut feeling. But industrial quality improvement experience (as well as that of the NDP) has shown that, in most cases, elaborate measures are not necessary. A simple, well-designed form that can be filled out with Xs or tally marks is often all that is required.

Designing the Data-Collection Form. The need for data can occur either when the team is *selecting and defining its problem, testing a theory about causes,* or *checking on the effectiveness of a solution.* Regardless of where the team is in its problem-solving journey, the design of a good data-collection form generally proceeds along the following lines:

- *What question* do we need to answer?
- *What data-analysis tools* (Pareto diagram, histogram, bar graph, and so on) do we envision using?
- *What type of data* do we need to construct this tool and answer the question?
- *Where* in the process can we get this data?
- *Who* in the process can give us this data?
- What is the *simplest format* in which to gather this data from these people?
- What *other (minimum) information* do we need to capture on the form for future reference and traceability?

As part of its effort to develop guidelines for the use of ultrasound tests, the Harvard Community Health Plan team needed data on the frequency of various indications (reasons for ordering the tests) in order to focus their resources on those indications that occurred most often. The team used the preceding questions to guide their design of an appropriate data-collection form:

- *Question of interest:* Which ultrasound test indications occur most frequently?
- *Analysis tool:* Pareto diagram.
- *Data needed:* Counts of tests by indication.
- *Where:* At the point when the tests are ordered.
- *Who:* Physician ordering test.
- *Simplest format:* Provide checklist of indications on order form.
- *Other information:* Patient information, physician information, further breakdown on some indications, any comments about special conditions.

Such a thorough process led to the development of the checklist shown in Exhibit B.8, which was the *instrument* for collecting the data that were to be displayed in the form of the Pareto diagram described earlier (see Exhibit B.5).

Simple data-collection forms, such as the one just described, were also used by other teams in the NDP at various stages in their problem-solving efforts:

Exhibit B.8. Data-Collection Form on Obstetrical Ultrasound (Harvard Community Health Plan Project).

Obstetrical Ultrasound Order Form

___ ___ ___ - ___ ___ - ___ ___
___
___ ___ / ___ ___ / ___ ___
EDC ___ ___ / ___ ___ / ___ ___ Urgency _____
___ ___ ___ ___ Ordering Provider _____

\#:

Name:

Center:

Date:

Reasons for Ordering Ultrasound (check one or more)

☐ Dating
☐ R/O IUGR or follow-up for IUGR ────►
☐ 1st trimester bleeding
☐ 2nd/3rd trimester bleeding.
☐ Large for Gestational Age/ Estimated Fetal Weight
☐ Fetal Survey
☐ Post dates/BPP
☐ Malposition
☐ BPP
☐ Other_____

If for IUGR (check primary reason)

☐ 1st U/S for R/O IUGR
☐ Follow-up U/S for IUGR
☐ BPP for IUGR
☐ Amniocentesis for IUGR
☐ BPP and Amniocentesis for IUGR

▼

if reason for Ultrasound is R/O or follow-up for IUGR please complete the following by checking the appropriate boxes:

☐ IUGr in a previous pregnancy
☐ Chronic hypertension
☐ Diabetes
☐ Malnutrition
☐ Alcohol/Drug Abuse
☐ Sever Bleeding in early pregnancy
☐ Abnormal AFP
☐ Other serious maternal diseases - SLE, cardiac, etc.
☐ Multiple Gestation
☐ Smoking, pregnancy induced hypertension, gestational diabetes
☐ Inadequate maternal weight gain
☐ "Small for dates"
☐ Fundal size assessment impossible (i.e. obesity, fibroids)
☐ Earler U/S for another reason indicates possible IUGR

Comments_____
_____

Please return this completed form to: Quality-of-Care Measurement. Hearthstone Plaza - 5th Floor 731-7575

- The University of Michigan Hospitals, North Carolina Memorial Hospital, and Beth Israel Hospital team used simple forms to tally the causes for discharge delays.
- The Park Nicollet team, looking into the causes for delays in telephone access based on the data displayed in Exhibit 7.3, asked receptionists and nurses to tally the type, number, and disposition of calls at the busiest hours.

A note of caution about data collection is in order here. While it is desirable to have all the data associated with a process problem, this is not always practical. Quality improvement teams must often rely on *sampling* from a representative time period or set of cases. Whenever samples are used, teams must take great care to assure that the sample is selected in a way that is representative of the larger population. (The statistical and practical considerations involved in selecting a sample are covered in most introductory statistical texts. See, for example, Sec. 25 of *Juran's Quality Control Handbook,* cited in Resource D.)

Graphs and Charts

The simple graphs and charts of industrial quality improvement are so generally useful, applicable, and easy to construct that it is hard to imagine a project that would not benefit from their use. Graphs and charts communicate much more information at a glance than do simple tables of numbers. Furthermore, as we will see in an example below, they are often far superior to a simple summary statistic such as an average.

Line graphs, bar graphs, and pie charts are the most familiar and commonly used tools for displaying data.

- *Line graphs* (also called *run charts*) are used to identify and display trends in data, typically trends over time.
- *Pie charts* are used to display information about the relative parts of a whole.
- *Bar graphs* are used to show comparisons among categorical data.

Line Graphs

The NDP team at Rhode Island Group Health Association used line graphs to analyze and display information about waiting times for appointments in their pediatrics department. The department had set a target of four to six weeks for appointment waiting times. The average waiting time for the ten-month period from October 1986 to July 1987 was about 4.6 weeks — seemingly on target.

But a line graph of the data, reproduced in Exhibit B.9, gives a very different picture from the average.

The left half of the graph (October 1986 to July 1987) shows that while the *average* of about 4.6 weeks is in the target zone, the *trend* in the data is clearly toward unacceptable waiting times. The summary statistic (the average) obscured the problem; the line graph made it clear.

Exhibit B.9 also illustrates another key point about how simple tools aid quality improvement by *helping a team monitor the condition of the process*. Note that there appears to be a new trend developing toward longer waiting times beginning in January 1988. This simple line graph is an efficient monitor of the performance of the process, providing an early warning of a potential recurrence of the problem after the solution has been implemented.

Histograms

While the common bar graph is used to display data that fall into categories, the histogram (or frequency distribution chart) is a special type of bar chart used to display the variation in continuous data like time, weight, size, or temperature.

We know that values in a set of data will almost always show variation. For example, the time required to move patients from the emergency room to a floor bed varies from patient to patient, depending on factors such as the availability of transport personnel, the patient's condition, or whether the elevators are working properly. This variation is also evident in critical measures such as blood count, pulse rate, or amount of anesthesia required.

Exhibit B.9. Waiting Times in Pediatrics (Rhode Island Group Health Association Project).

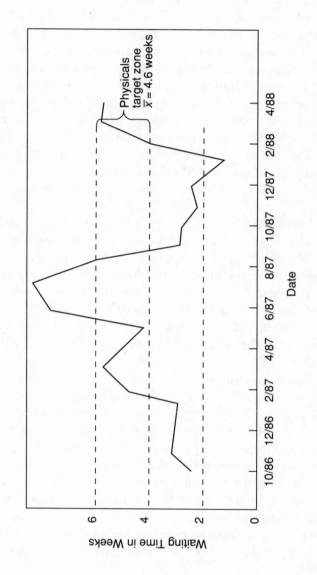

In most cases, this inherent variation is unpredictable on an event-by-event basis. For instance, we cannot say beforehand exactly how long it will take to move a patient, what a patient's blood count or pulse rate will be, or precisely how much anesthesia will be needed. But this inherent variation *does* typically follow some pattern. We might say, for example, that "it takes thirty minutes on average to move a patient; it never takes less than fifteen minutes, but sometimes it can take up to two hours" or "given the patient's weight and condition, anesthesia should take between *X* and *Y* minutes." In statistical terminology, these patterns are called *distributions.*

The histogram is a graphic tool that enables a quality improvement team to analyze these patterns of distributions in data—patterns that are typically not apparent by simply looking at the table of data.

In the NDP, the team from Worcester Memorial used histograms to study variation in the response time of the hospital's laboratory to physicians' orders for laboratory work on emergency department patients. The team's report clearly outlines the systematic use of the tools of quality improvement as the team proceeds on its "diagnostic journey": "The group first developed a *flow diagram* of the current process now in place between the time when a physician writes an order . . . and when the test results are available. Next, a *cause-and-effect diagram* was drawn. These two graphical tools allowed the group to identify two problem areas which warranted more detailed study. The first problem area dealt with the transport of specimens from the emergency department to the laboratory, and the second dealt with the processing of a specimen after it had been received in the laboratory. *Data were collected* with regard to the second problem area, over a 12-day period. . . . These data were then arrayed on a *run chart* [line graph], *a histogram,* and on *control charts* [see next section]. . . . The data, charts, and diagrams, along with the discussion they evoked, resulted in . . . recommendations . . . which have been implemented."

Exhibit B.10 shows the 100 measurements made by the team of actual laboratory response times.

Exhibit B.10. Laboratory Response Times (Minutes), Evening Shift: Tabular Form (Worcester Memorial Hospital Project).

11	13	15	17	17	18	18	19	19	20
20	20	20	20	20	21	21	21	21	22
22	22	22	22	23	23	23	23	23	23
24	24	24	24	25	25	25	26	26	26
26	26	26	27	27	27	27	27	28	28
28	28	28	28	28	28	29	29	30	30
31	31	31	32	33	33	33	33	34	34
35	35	35	35	36	37	37	37	38	38
39	39	42	45	46	46	47	48	48	49
50	50	51	52	53	53	53	54	55	62

Although Exhibit B.10 contains a great deal of additional information about the variation in response times, it is difficult to extract that information from the list of numbers alone. Much more can be learned when the same data are displayed in the form of a histogram. The histogram of the laboratory's response time during the evening shift is shown in Exhibit B.11. The height of each bar indicates the frequency with which the response time fell within that time interval. The numbers on the horizontal axis indicate the midpoint of the time interval. For example, the histogram shows that twenty-four specimens had processing times that fell in the interval from 24.5 to 29.5 minutes (midpoint 27 minutes).

Note the variation in response times. Of more interest than the frequency of response times in any one interval is the *overall pattern* that the histogram reveals. For example, the team can now see clearly that:

- The variation in response time is wide, ranging from about ten minutes to about an hour.
- The majority of specimens were processed in twenty to thirty minutes.
- The distribution is not symmetrical; there are very few response times less than twenty minutes, but many that are greater than thirty minutes (in other words, the distribution is "skewed").

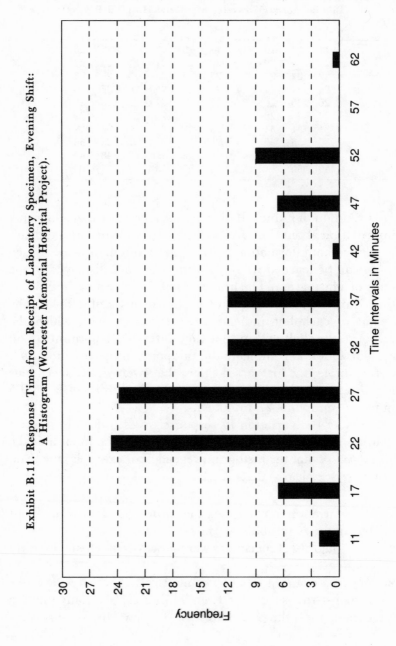

Exhibit B.11. Response Time from Receipt of Laboratory Specimen, Evening Shift: A Histogram (Worcester Memorial Hospital Project).

- The distribution appears to have two peaks: one around twenty-five minutes and another around fifty minutes (indicating that not *one*, but *two* processes may actually be at work).

Histograms are commonly used in this way by quality improvement teams *to characterize a situation* and *identify areas for further data analysis.*

The team from Children's Hospital used histograms in their study of the time associated with transporting critically ill infants and children from referring hospitals into their tertiary care facility. They used a variant of the histogram called the *stem-and-leaf plot,* first suggested by statistician John Tukey. The plot in Exhibit B.12 shows the distribution of time between a call from a referring facility and the departure of the special transport team from Children's Hospital.

Exhibit B.12. Elapsed Time Between Call and Departure of Team:
A Stem-and-Leaf Plot (Children's Hospital Project).

2*	000
2.	5
3*	
3.	555558
4*	00
4.	55557
5*	0000000000002
5.	5555555555
6*	0000
6.	5555555
7*	000000
7.	55
8*	00
8.	5
9*	000
9.	5

2* 0 represents 20 minutes

Stem-and-leaf plots differ from traditional histograms in that they cleverly retain a great deal of the original numerical data that histograms lose. In the stem-and-leaf plot, the bars of the traditional histogram are replaced by a string of digits. To construct a stem-and-leaf plot, one first writes the major divisions (the numbers to the left of the decimals in Exhibit B.12) in a column. The rows of numbers in Exhibit B.12 indicate time in five-minute intervals; the time intervals range from 20 (2* 0) to 95 (9. 5) minutes. Each observation is noted by writing the final digit of the observation on the same line as the major division. For example, the observation of 45 minutes would be entered by going to the "4." line and writing the numeral "5" on that line; an observation of 70 minutes is indicated by the numeral "0" on the "7*" line; 52 minutes is a "2" on the "5*" line; and so on. (Reading the plot from the top, we see that there were three observations of 20 minutes, one of 25, none between 30 and 34, five of 35, one of 38, and so on.) The result is a histogram displaying a pattern of variation. Technically, stem-and-leaf plots have an advantage over the traditional bar-form histogram (like the one in Exhibit B.11) in that *they preserve the identity of each individual observation,* although neither histograms nor stem-and-leaf plots preserve the *order* in which the data were collected.

The resulting diagram enabled the team from Children's Hospital to analyze the patterns in the data, characterize the situation, and identify areas for further exploration. The team noted that in approximately 95 percent of the cases, it took at least thirty-five minutes for the special transport personnel to leave the hospital. Comparing this distribution to those for other phases of the overall transport process, the team noted that this "in-house" time represented more than 50 percent of the total time in about 75 percent of the cases. The team had used data collection and histogram (stem-and-leaf) display in order to localize the problem; they proceeded to focus their energies on developing and testing theories about the causes for these in-house delays.

Simple histograms, like the examples shown here, are important tools for analyzing data on the continuous variables that commonly occur in the health care setting (for example, time, medication dosage, laboratory results). We know that such measures will have inherent variation, but *the pattern of that variation is usually not evident in a simple table of the data.* Furthermore, summary statistics such as the average do not tell us everything about the pattern. For example, the average laboratory response time in Exhibit B.11 is about thirty-one minutes. But this statement alone does not tell us about the small additional peak at around fifty minutes, nor does it tell us that the response times can be as high as an hour. The histogram tells a much richer story than the summary statistics do.

Control Charts and Other Analytical Methods

The histogram is a basic, visual tool for analyzing variation. The science of statistics has also provided more sophisticated analytical techniques for the use of quality managers. These tools, such as control charts, hypothesis tests, regression analysis, correlation analysis, and analysis of variance (ANOVA), have helped in industrial quality improvement efforts. Many of these, too, found application in the NDP.

Control charts were developed in the 1920s by Walter Shewhart, a pioneer in industrial quality control, to help managers and workers reduce the costs of inspection and rejection and to attain uniform quality. Control charts are based on the concept that some variation is inherent in any process. More specifically, control chart theory recognizes that there is inherent variation in repeated measurements from a process, *even if the process itself does not change.* (Our discussion of control chart theory here is simplified. The interested reader can refer to the texts cited in Resource D for more detail.)

A quality improvement team needs a way to distinguish between variation that derives from the inherent properties of the process being studied (plus random variation in the measurements used to study it) and the variation that comes from real and significant *changes* in the process. The former is called "common cause variation," while the latter is referred to as "special cause variation." *The control chart is the tool for helping the user*

determine if a process can be considered stable and thus predictable, or
unstable and thus unpredictable.

A control chart from the report of the Worcester Memorial team is shown in Exhibit B.13. (The $\bar{X}$ chart is shown alone, without the usual accompanying R chart. For details of types of control charts, see the texts referenced in Resource D.)

The graph shows the average time delay in discharging patients (freeing up a bed) after the physician's orders are written. The dotted line labeled "$\bar{\bar{X}}$" (read: "X double-bar") shows the average of these daily averages. The lines labeled "UCL" and "LCL" show the upper and lower control limits, respectively. These control limits are calculated based on statistical theory and represent the range of variation inherent in the process, that is, common cause variation. That range is estimated from the data themselves, using rules developed by Shewhart and the theorists who followed him. Points that fall outside of the control limits indicate a high probability that the process was truly different on those days; in other words, a special cause of variation is probably present and a true process shift has occurred. (In addition to points that fall outside the limits, certain other trends in the patterns of points within the limits can also indicate special causes of variation. See sec. 24 of *Juran's Quality Control Handbook,* cited in Resource D.)

From the control chart in Exhibit B.13, the team was able to derive the following observations and conclusions:

- Because they fall within the control limits, days 1,2,4,6,7, and 8 must be considered "typical." The variability in discharge times on these days is not significant enough to warrant detailed investigation of special causes of variation. All values likely represent properties of the process itself.
- Days 3 and 5 had significantly longer discharge times, probably due to special influences *not* part of the usual process. (We are greatly oversimplifying control chart theory here. A more rigorous examination of this chart, and the associated R chart, shows that the difference on day 7 is also statistically significant.) The team must now ask: Why? What happened on those days that would make them different?

Exhibit B.13. Admission Process Time from M.D. Order to Actual ER Discharge: A Control Chart – $\bar{X}$ Chart (Worcester Memorial Hospital Project).

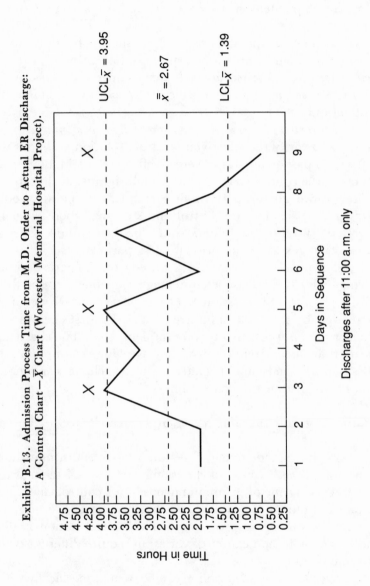

- Day 9 had significantly shorter discharge times, another "special cause" variation. Again, the team must ask: Why? What happened on this day that would make it different?

As this example illustrates, the addition of control limits is a critical enhancement to the standard line graph. *The control limits enable a team to sort out and classify causes of variation in the data.* Operationally, this helps focus the team's subsequent investigation.

The control chart is also an important tool for monitoring a process in order to verify the effectiveness of the solution and hold the gains from past quality improvement efforts. If a solution is truly effective, the control chart should show a significant shift in the process toward better performance, that is, data points should begin falling outside the control limits on the "good" side. In effect, the intervention should introduce systematic, "special cause" changes from the prior process performance.

The team from Park Nicollet used control charts as monitoring tools to help them better manage telephone access in their family practice unit. Exhibit B.14 compares the "average time to answer" by the medical information (MI) nurses before and after process improvements were implemented. The charts indicate that "mean time to answer" was reduced from 208 seconds to 103 seconds, and that after the process changes answering times were within the control limits.

Tampering and the Theory of Statistical Process Control

We have made much of the importance of distinguishing *special* from *common* causes of variation in processes. Making such a distinction is one of the main purposes of a control chart. Let us take a moment to examine *why* that distinction is so crucial to effective quality improvement. The central notion is that special and common causes of variation require different types of remedy.

Special causes of variation can be treated specifically without modifying the basic, underlying process. When the Park Nicollet team discovered that pulling receptionists away from

their jobs to be trained caused highly unusual increases in telephone response times, they were able to recommend a change
in training schedules. The cause of the poor phone response was
specific, evident, and *not* part of the "routine" phone answering
process. Juran uses the term "attributable variation" in place
of "special cause" to emphasize this aspect of variation of this
type.

By contrast, "common cause" variation (Juran calls it "random variation") cannot be explained by citing influences outside the process itself. The variation is a *property* of the process,
just like the *average* performance level. The underlying reasons
for this common, random variation are numerous, nonspecific,
obscure, and, without a fundamental change in the process itself,
inevitable. (Actually, one other source of common cause variation is the way we *measure* the process. All real measurements
have some random component of error, and this error is present
in any graph or number we use to describe a process.)

If we find that a process has only common cause variation in it, which we can determine using some statistical rules
contributed by Shewhart and those who followed him, we can
say that the process is, by definition, "in statistical control." This
is not to say that the process "performs well," but only that it
is stable and thus predictable; special causes of variation are
not in evidence. Because the process is stable, it is meaningful
to ask about its average performance level, or its "capability."
At Park Nicollet, the average "capability" of the "receptionist
phone answering process" (after the special cause variation was
removed) seemed to be around thirty-seven seconds.

What if we are dissatisfied with the process capability of
a stable process? Say, for example, that telephone callers *still*
complain frequently about delayed service even when the phone
answering process is in statistical control, with a mean answering time of thirty-seven seconds. In that case, without special
causes to treat, we are left with only one option for improvement: *to change the process itself.* If we go about "treating" the random variation by intervening specifically when answering times
appear to be high (but not high enough to be of special cause),
we may make things worse. "Treating" random variation only

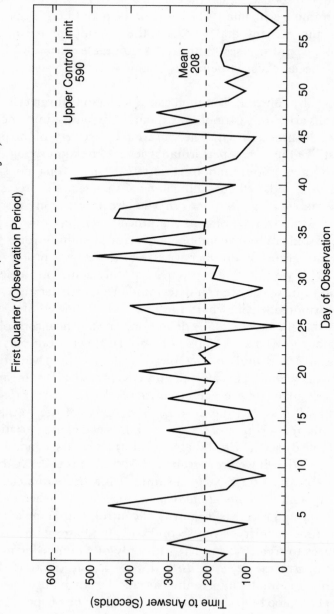

Exhibit B.14. Average Time for Medical Information Nurses to Answer Telephone Between 9:00 and 10:00 A.M. (Park Nicollet Project).

Exhibit B.14. Average Time for Medical Information Nurses to Answer Telephone Between 9:00 and 10:00 A.M. (Park Nicollet Project), Cont'd.

Month of April (Postintervention)

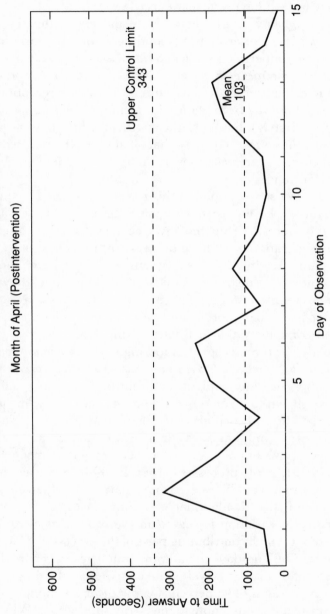

increases the variation, and we can fool ourselves into thinking that we are having a real effect.

Quality control engineers use the term "tampering" to refer to two kinds of error in responding to process variation. One type of tampering is *treating special causes of variation as if they were inherent properties of the process.* That is overreacting, and it makes little logical sense. It is one thing to ask that receptionists not be pulled away from phones for training (treating special cause appropriately), but it is quite another to change the *whole process* (for example, by requiring that all absences be reduced) simply because, on rare occasions, training has interfered with process performance.

We see examples of this type of tampering frequently in medicine. In one recent case, an error was made by a referring doctor in reading a pathology specimen, leading to an unnecessary operation. The hospital's response was to require repeat, in-house readings of all specimens of all types, even though the hospital administrators could not possibly have known if the index event was of special cause or not. They may well have tampered with a process, and thereby introduced waste, rework, and complexity that will later haunt them.

The other type of tampering is *to treat common cause variation as if it were special.* This happens when a supervisor requires a subordinate to "explain" an event that a control chart would have shown to be merely random, and not really "explainable" as the effect of a single, identifiable cause.

Imagine that X-ray images are inadequate and require repeat views on the average five percent of the time in an X-ray unit with stable processes. From day to day, the actual repeat rates might vary between two percent and ten percent, not because of special, identifiable circumstances, but because that degree of variation is *inherent* in the process as a result of the dozens of small contributing parts of the process of taking X-rays there. On Tuesday, the administrator gets a report that nine percent of all X-rays were retaken, whereas the proportion has been averaging five percent for the prior six months. The administrator sends a note to the X-ray supervisor: "Why was the retake rate so high on Tuesday?"

What happens next is merely waste. The supervisor goes about collecting opinions and explanations from the X-ray staff, formulates a theory of the reason, and reports back to the administrator. Perhaps the supervisor concludes that the temperature in the film storage area *may* have been too hot that day. The administrator asks the building services manager to look into it. And so it goes: busy people wasting their time "fixing" a special problem that never existed at all. Since the next retake rate may well be lower (random variation is like that), the people involved may even feel good about their time-wasting tampering. They fixed the "blame" for a random blip up, and they take the "credit" for the next random blip down.

Tampering wastes time, increases complexity, and obscures real opportunities to make processes better. The control chart, which helps draw clear distinctions between special and common causes of variation, is the best medicine against the ills of tampering.

Hypothesis Testing

Teams in the NDP also applied other statistical analysis techniques in their quality improvement efforts. One such technique, *hypothesis testing*—which is widely used in health care to evaluate data from controlled experiments on the efficacy of different treatment techniques—is closely related to the control chart technique described earlier. Hypothesis-testing techniques are typically used to determine the significance of differences when a team has only two measurements, while control charts are used to analyze a continuing series of measurements.

The team from Presbyterian Hospital used hypothesis tests at the end of the "remedial journey," to determine whether the guidelines they had developed for the use of portable X-rays were having a significant impact on the frequency of inappropriate use. Following a simple experimental protocol commonly used by design and manufacturing engineers in the industrial setting, the team first did a retrospective study of thirty patients' charts to determine the percentage of inappropriate use *before* the guidelines were introduced. Then the team distributed the guidelines and again measured the percentage of inappropriate portable X-rays.

The question the team wanted to answer was, "Did the guidelines help reduce the percentage of inappropriate portable X-rays?" But since the measurements were done on a sample, the team knew intuitively that it was possible, due to random variation, for the calculated "after" percentage to be less than the "before" percentage, *even if the guidelines had had no effect.* Therefore, the team used hypothesis tests to determine if the "after" percentage was significantly better than the "before" percentage.

In a hypothesis test, one begins by assuming that there is no real difference between "before" and "after." This is called the "null hypothesis." The test involves calculating the probability of seeing the observed result if this null hypothesis is true. If that probability is low, we reject the null hypothesis and conclude that a significant difference *does* exist.

The Presbyterian Hospital team used the binomial distribution to calculate the probabilities associated with the null hypothesis (in this case, that the guidelines had had no effect). The binomial distribution is a well-known mathematical relationship for calculating the probability of r occurrences of an event in n (in this case, 30) samples. The resulting calculations showed that there was less than a .05 chance that the null hypothesis was true. Rather, it was highly likely that the "after" percentage was better than the "before" percentage and that the guidelines had indeed had a positive impact on performance.

In addition to control charts and formal hypothesis testing, teams in the NDP also used other, more advanced statistical analysis techniques. Teams from UCLA and the University of Michigan, for example, used scatter plots and regression and correlation analysis to study the causal relationships between factors in the processes of outpatient appointments and hospital discharge. The Johns Hopkins team designed a relatively sophisticated experiment and planned to use analysis-of-variance (ANOVA) methods to distinguish the variation due to sampling from that due to true differences in the relative effectiveness of many different preanesthesia screening processes. Though these more technically complex methods definitely have a place in quality improvement, the simpler tools are certainly powerful enough for most teams to gain extraordinary new insights into processes and variation.

Summary and Future Directions

The National Demonstration Project on Quality Improvement in Health Care achieved its goal of showing that the concepts and tools of industrial quality improvement can be used to improve the quality of processes in the health care industry. Process flow diagrams, Pareto diagrams, cause-and-effect diagrams, histograms, control charts, and so on — the familiar tools of industrial quality improvement — were successfully applied to a wide variety of health care processes.

In using the tools, the health care teams found what those in other industries have also found. The tools themselves are not difficult to use; the key ingredients that quality management offers are leadership, involvement, dedication to a problem-solving discipline, and the *opportunity* to use systematic tools to learn about processes.

Resource C:
Three Project Reports

Kaiser-Permanente Medical Care Program Follow-Up Care: Improving Records Transfers for Greater Efficiency and Effectiveness*

Kaiser-Permanente Medical Care Program, Northern California

Introduction

When a medical center patient appears for follow-up care after hospital emergency treatment, and the emergency department (ED) record is not at hand, the quality of care can be affected. In a certain number of cases, therefore, the physicians will not proceed without making every effort to obtain the ED record. The patient cannot always be relied on for the information needed for appropriate care; not uncommonly, patients even fail to mention that they had been treated for an emergency.

Without the ED records, the physicians must get the data by phoning the ED, which prolongs the visit and may aggravate everyone involved including the patient. Correcting for lack of data is costly in physician time and in staff time at the ED

*By Robert Formanek, M.D., Assistant Director of Quality; Leonard Rubin, M.D., Director of Quality; and Bruce J. Sams, Jr., M.D., Executive Director.

221

records room. The delays of other waiting patients can lead to backups, rescheduling, and patient dissatisfaction. In a system the size of the Kaiser-Permanente Medical Care Program (KPMCP) in Northern California, the cumulative effects of lost physician time and patient delays can be substantial.

The KPMCP in Northern California consists of fourteen Kaiser-Foundation Hospitals with adjoining ambulatory facilities (medical centers) and an additional twelve medical office buildings. The program serves over 2 million Kaiser-Permanente Foundation Health Plan members, as well as a substantial number of patients who have other health care payment arrangements. There are 2,700 physicians and 21,000 other personnel.

The site selected for the KPMCP National Demonstration Project was the Santa Clara Medical Center (SCL) and its two associated medical office buildings, one in Sunnyvale (SUN) and the other in Milpitas (MIL). These three facilities surround the southern end of San Francisco Bay, and make up the Santa Clara service area. Santa Clara Medical Center is 6 miles from Sunnyvale and 13 miles from Milpitas. Health care is provided for approximately 230,430 members within this service area.

Santa Clara itself provides medical offices for 187 physicians, while Milpitas and Sunnyvale provide medical offices for thirty-six and nineteen physicians, respectively. KPMCP members are free to visit any of the delivery sites in the Northern California region and often use two or more facilities.

The Project

When Drs. Berwick and Godfrey invited the Northern California KPMCP to participate in the National Demonstration Project, this invitation was recognized by top management as an opportunity to be embraced. The program takes pride in having been a pioneer in quality assurance in health care. For the past two decades the KPMCP in Northern California has used the concepts embodied in the comprehensive quality assurance system (CQAS) as its primary approach to quality improvement. The invitation was perceived as a research opportunity to enhance CQAS and our other quality control and quality improvement activities. The expectations were to gain insights and to learn and apply new techniques from the non–health care industry. These expectations were realized through the use of modalities such as process flow diagrams, cause-effect diagrams, Pareto diagrams, internal as well as external customer distinctions, and process performance measurements.

Project Selection

The problem originally selected by the KPMCP in Northern California for the National Demonstration Project was the timely transfer of clinical data from medical centers to their satellite medical office buildings. After due consideration, the scope of the issue was recognized to be too broad. Major progress in selection occurred when the project was narrowed. It was limited to one medical center, the Kaiser-Permanente Santa Clara Medical Center (SCL) with its two satellites, Milpitas (MIL) and Sunnyvale (SUN).

Furthermore, the group assembled to work on the issue (the physician-in-chief, physicians-in-charge, facility administrators, and selected department heads from SCL, SUN, and MIL) narrowed it to one particular area of clinical information transfer that was especially bothersome to staff and patients: "the timely transfer of appropriate emergency department clinical data from SCL to its two satellites, MIL and SUN."

Project Team

The individuals working on the problem were divided into two groups, the steering committee and the working group. The steering committee included the physicians-in-chief from each of the three facilities, the SCL medical center administrator, and the SCL administrative assistant who coordinated the project. The working group was composed of the SCL administrative assistant, the medical office building administrators from MIL and SUN, the chartroom supervisors from all three locations, the SCL reception supervisor, the SCL emergency reception supervisor, and the SCL emergency head nurse. The director and assistant director of quality from the Permanente Medical Group, Inc. (TPMG) attended meetings of both groups, as did the quality manager from Hewlett-Packard who coordinated the project.

Identifying Causes

The issue proved to be more difficult and complex than first anticipated. Patients are free to visit any of the Kaiser-Permanente offices, and some regularly visit all three sites for a variety of reasons. Emergency care is commonly sought and delivered at the site nearest the patient when the emergency occurs. Often this is not the location usually visited by the patient or the location of the patient's regular physician. In other cases where the patient's condition is serious, or when emergency care is sought after medical office building hours, it will be obtained at the SCL emergency department, since this is the one site with hospital beds and with twenty-four-hour emergency services.

Clarifying the Process

The site for follow-up care of patients who were seen at the SCL emergency department had been determined by the ED receptionist, based on patients' answering questions or volunteering the information.

Several problems with this step in the process were immediately apparent: When the ED was very busy, the receptionists did not have time to get the information. Patients under stress, or because of language barriers, gave erroneous answers. At least one receptionist expected patients to volunteer the information because a sign on the wall asked that they do so.

Another step in this process was the sorting of all copies of the SCL emergency visit data. This sorting included the copies designated for transfer to SUN and MIL. Through this sorting procedure copies were selected for distribution to several SCL in-house departments including pediatrics, obstetrics and gynecology, ophthalmology, and allergy. Distribution of the emergency visit data to the SCL departments was given priority over distribution to SUN and MIL, and this significantly diluted the number of records eventually sent to the medical offices.

The process of *transferring* emergency visit data to the medical office buildings was initially assessed by measuring the frequency of appropriate and timely distribution of clinical information from the emergency visits. A frequency distribution over time was analyzed to learn more of the magnitude and character of the problem and to assist in analysis of the process flow diagram.

Lessons from the Flow Diagrams

At the first meeting of the working group, a process flow diagram was constructed. This was referred to and revised periodically as new information surfaced and as progress was made toward solving the problem. An important element fell into place when one of the members of the working group declared "ownership" of the process. Existing process performance measurements validated the perception that emergency visit records were not getting into the medical office building charts. A cause-and-effect diagram was used to represent suspected and known flaws in the process, and various customer needs and expectations were established.

In analysis of flow diagrams (Exhibits C.1 and C.2), much was learned about the process that had not been realized. Continuing analysis followed with additional measurements as refinements, and changes in the process flow diagram occurred concomitant with revelations about the actual process.

The actual process was far from that originally perceived by any of the working group members. Exhibits C.1 and C.2 illustrate the original and a subsequent flow diagram. This demonstrates how different the initial perception of the process was from the actual. The analytic process revealed unnecessary delivery of information to some departments and satellites and inadequate delivery to others. During this time the actual information needs of the clinical departments and of the medical office buildings (all internal customers) were clarified and reclarified.

Exhibit C.1. Initial Description of Record Transfer Process:
A Process Flow Diagram (Kaiser-Permanente Project).

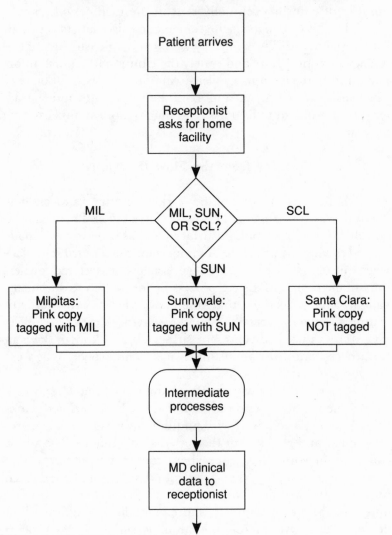

Exhibit C.1. Initial Description of Record Transfer Process:
A Process Flow Diagram (Kaiser-Permanente Project), Cont'd.

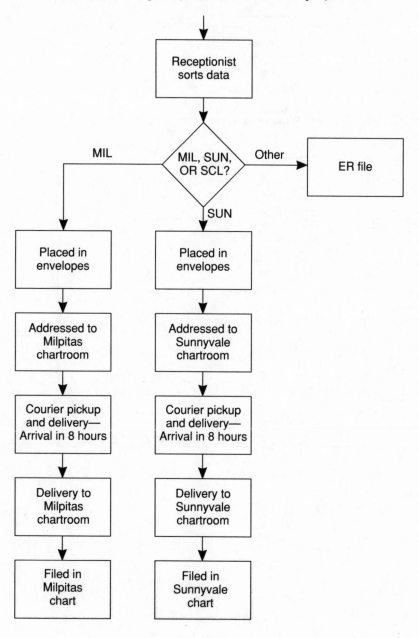

**Exhibit C.2. Revised Description of Record Transfer Process:
A Process Flow Diagram (Kaiser-Permanente Project).**

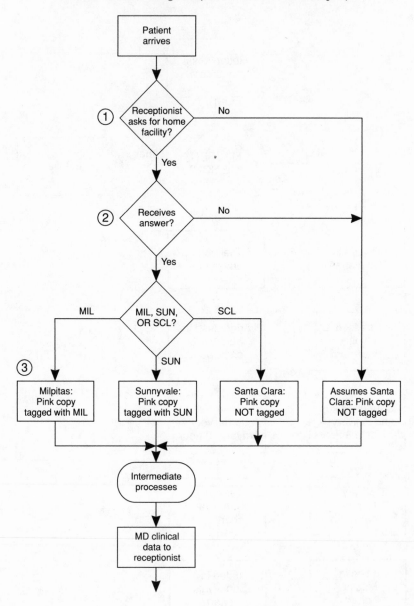

Exhibit C.2. Revised Description of Record Transfer Process:
A Process Flow Diagram (Kaiser-Permanente Project), Cont'd.

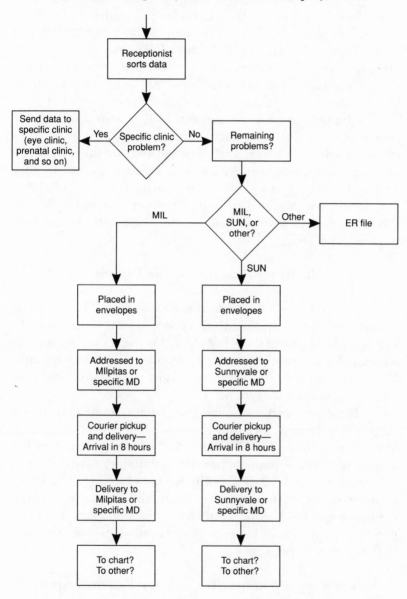

Cause-and-Effect Diagram

In addition to the above, errors in the delivery process were discovered, and these were modified and corrected almost immediately on discovery. Exhibit C.3 demonstrates by means of a cause-and-effect diagram some of the problems discovered. Continued analysis and measurement followed, using the number of visits reported and received and the transit time.

The primary cause identified as a system flaw was the *patient-inquiry method* for determining the site of the patient's follow-up care. However, analysis indicated that the system was not likely to succeed even with modifications in patient inquiry and in the sorting and handling of records. It was decided that a major system change was needed in order to have the desired records available at the location where the patient would subsequently be seen.

Remedy—Improving the Process

The obvious solution to this problem would seem to be a computerized central medical records system. However, the size and complexity of the KPMCP in Northern California make it unsuitable for existing computerized medical records systems. Nor did the budget for the project allow us to design and construct a new records system.

However, various online computer systems exist in the KPMCP in Northern California. One of these contains an up-to-date inventory (chart inventory) of where each patient has a medical chart. A patient chart for ambulatory care is created whenever a patient visits a facility for the first time. These ambulatory care charts are kept by the medical office adjacent to the hospital or by the satellite medical office buildings. The computer chart inventory for each patient indicates where an ambulatory care chart exists.

Substituting Computer Inquiry for Patient Inquiry

With this in mind, we decided that within twenty-four hours of the time of a visit to the SCL emergency department

Exhibit C.3. Cause-and-Effect Diagram for Timely Transfer of Emergency Room Records to Satellite Medical Office Building (Kaiser-Permanente Project).

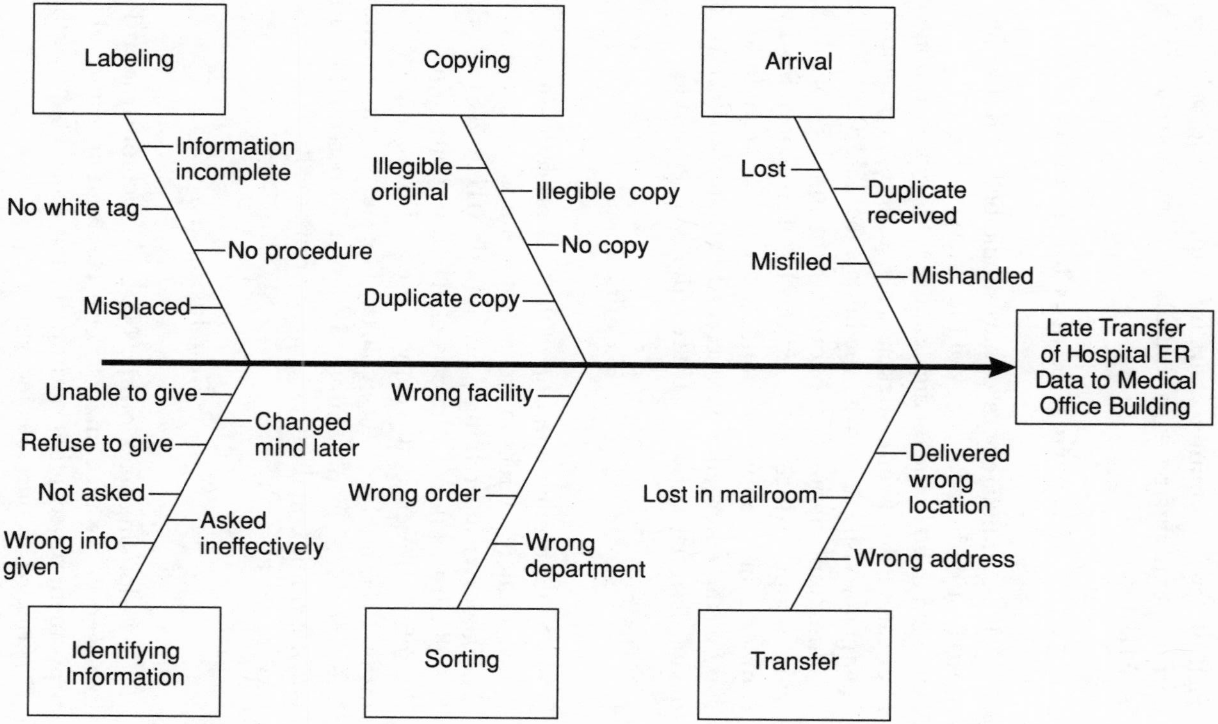

each patient's computer chart inventory would be accessed to permit identifying patients' ambulatory care charts in SUN and/ or MIL.

Preparing Records for Transfer

If an ambulatory care chart should be found in either SUN or MIL or both, then a copy of the emergency visit record would be tagged to go to the medical office(s). "Tagging" is done by the application of a white sticker tag to a designated copy of the emergency visit record with the initials "MIL," "SUN," or "SCL," or some combination of the three written on the white tag. This white tag procedure is carried out by all receptionists over the course of the twenty-four hours from 9:00 A.M. to 9:00 A.M. A copy of the emergency visit record is then transferred to each of the designated locales by routine courier service.

Results

Since implementation of the new process, there has been approximately a tenfold increase in the number of copies of SCL emergency visits arriving daily at both MIL and SUN. Exhibit C.4 illustrates the results of a chart audit done to measure for the timely presence of a copy of the SCL emergency visit data in the MIL medical office charts. The success rate is shown to have increased from around 13 to over 70 percent (see Exhibit C.5). Exhibit C.6 illustrates more dramatically the effects of intervention at both sites.

Conclusion

In looking back on the National Demonstration Project experience, we recognize several elements in the quality improvement process that permitted us to achieve a breakthrough with regard to our selected issue.

Both the steering committee and the working group meetings and activities were facilitated by Debra Shenk of Hewlett-Packard, who was our mentor and partner, as was Dr. Frederick

Exhibit C.4. Presence of Emergency Data in Medical Office Charts (Kaiser-Permanente Project).

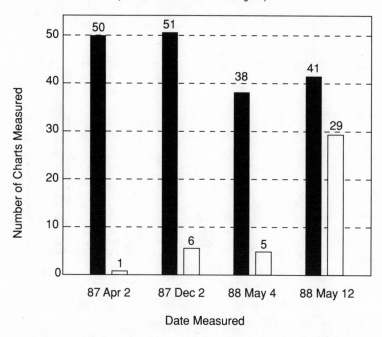

Mosteller of the Harvard University School of Public Health. This strong facilitation was certainly central to the purpose and the success of the project. If this project is an accurate model, then the quality improvement process is sustained by effective facilitation of the various groups involved.

There was a clear and distinct message from local management that this issue would be fully engaged and resolved. Appropriate resources in the form of work session time, information gathering assignments, and additional receptionist time were authorized. This provided a sense of empowerment for the working group and reinforced their determination to succeed. It also resulted in the collection of information that was necessary for a detailed account of each of the actual steps of the processes involved.

Exhibit C.5. Santa Clara Emergency Room Records: Milpitas Charts
(Kaiser-Permanente Project).

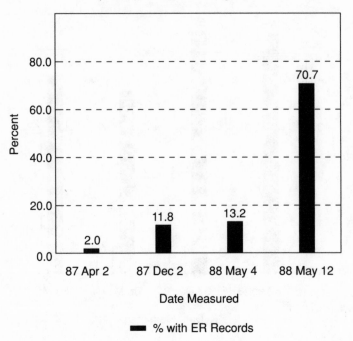

As previously noted, the first major progress occurred when the project scope was narrowed to a manageable size. This made the project "doable" within realistic time and resource constraints. At the same time, the problem and its resolution remained illustrative of many of the aspects of the larger concern—that is, the original, more generalized issue.

An important step toward a solution was the declaration of "ownership" of the process by a member of the working group, the hospital reception supervisor. Also notable was the consistent representation from each facility at each meeting, which allowed the group to stay in communication about the facts and to clear up misconceptions. Equally important, the group developed a sense of mutual trust and respect for each other.

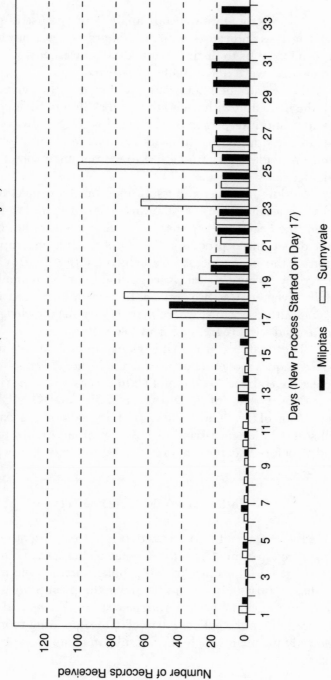

Exhibit C.6. Effects of Intervention on the Presence of Emergency Data in Medical Office Charts (Kaiser-Permanente Project).

The augmentation of our analysis by the use of process flow diagrams and cause-and-effect diagrams was considerable. These allowed us to distinguish additional elements within the process that were not initially recognized.

The group members were motivated in their interaction with the issue and with each other and skillful in their communications and interpersonal relationships. Of note was the fact that no one dominated the work sessions, and members were able to provide information and to express their views clearly and succinctly.

Middle managers and staff took on the project actively and were accountable for planning, coordinating, and carrying out the necessary actions. This culminated in the redesign of the data transfer process and its implementation. Implementation of the new process was helped by the "buy in" of the emergency reception staff. Recognition by management of the staff involvement was also notable. In part, this occurred at steering committee sessions, where management acknowledged and encouraged the progress as it unfolded into success.

The quality control and quality improvement methods and techniques modeled and used in the National Demonstration Project have already been applied to several different issues in other delivery sites of the Northern California KPMCP. The assimilation of these new activities seems to be working extremely well so far; a longer period of observation and more data are needed before a determination can be made of the degree of success.

Potential for Future Projects

In the wake of the success of this project, intentions have been voiced in Santa Clara to carry the techniques and methodology learned into other known problem areas. One problem specifically targeted in Santa Clara is the prompt availability of the chart, including all relevant laboratory, X-ray, and clinical information, on the patient's arrival in the operating room. This is a costly problem which often results in delay or cancellation of surgery.

These same methods and techniques have been introduced in Martinez Kaiser Foundation Hospital and Antioch medical office building where a working group has convened to improve the timely availability of consultation reports for the referring Antioch physician. Also on their agenda are timely transfer of emergency data and of discharge date to Antioch. Similar efforts exist in the Stockton and Fresno medical offices where difficulty has been recognized in obtaining various reports from outside facilities.

It remains to be seen whether these quality improvement methods will be replicated in other facilities. The extent to which we expand and share this quality improvement technology will be a test of the impact of this single project. If others are able to "stand on the shoulders" of the first group, to learn, and to carry the learning forward so as to similarly improve other and more varied issues, then the most meaningful objective will have been met.

Massachusetts General Hospital
Medicare Billing: Improving the Process
for Cost Reduction and Revenue Increases*

Massachusetts General Hospital, Boston

With ever-mounting regulatory constraints and unpredict-able reimbursement pressures continuing to threaten the finan-cial stability of health care providers, the need for an adaptable, accurate, and prompt billing system has never been more vital for hospitals. With these issues in mind, Massachusetts General Hospital (MGH) chose to investigate its Medicare inpatient bill-ing system as an area for potential quality improvement.

This issue has become particularly significant since the elimination of Medicare Periodic Interim Payments (PIP) in July 1987. Before the elimination of PIP, automatic monthly payments were made by Medicare regardless of the actual claims billed, with a year-end settlement process reflective of actual activity.

Defects in the billing system were sheltered by this earlier payment scheme. With the elimination of the shelter, the im-portance of producing an accurate and timely claim became a significant factor in the cash flow of the institution.

In fiscal year 1987, Medicare accounted for 34 percent of the discharged patients and 39 percent of net patient service revenue for MGH. The inability to produce a consistently ac-curate bill for Medicare services within a reasonable time after the patient is discharged has a severely negative impact on the institution's cash flow position.

Baseline.   To attach a dollar value to the problems of inaccurate and delayed claims, the month of November 1987

---

*By George P. Baker, Jr., M.D., Associate General Director for Medical Affairs; John Mahoney, Associate Director of Fiscal Affairs; Ann Prestipino, Director of Patient Services; James F. Riley, Jr., Vice President, Juran Institute, Inc.; Elizabeth Bradley, Administrative Fellow; William Kent, Administrative Fellow.

was used as a sample time period. During this time, the expected payment dollar value (gross charges less contractual adjustments) of all Medicare rejections at MGH was approximately $960,000. This includes backlogged rejected claims six months or older and current rejects. The majority of these rejected claims were ultimately paid by Medicare or another third-party payer after rebilling.

The process of correcting and resubmitting rejected claims delays cash flow for as long as three months. Assuming an average expected payment of $6,000 per claim and an interest rate of 8 percent, the cost due to delayed cash flow was approximately $120 per inaccurate claim, or $19,200 for the November 1987 baseline.

In addition to the cost of inaccuracies, there are long delays between the time the patient is discharged and the time the bill is sent to Medicare. Ideally, the lapse between discharge and billing is targeted at eight days. In our sample month, however, only half of the Medicare claims met this eight-day target. Furthermore, for those bills that were delayed longer than eight days, the average delay was seventeen to eighteen days, and 10 percent were delayed longer than thirty days before billing. The expected payment dollar value of the bills delayed longer than eight days after discharge was $1.62 million. Again assuming an 8 percent interest rate, the cash flow cost was $10,800 for the month.

If these combined problems of inaccurate and delayed billing of Medicare services persisted, the cost to MGH of delayed cash flow would total approximately $360,000 per year. An added cost is that for the additional personnel devoted to correcting inaccuracies and rebilling rejected claims. All rejected claims must be rebilled manually by MGH personnel and processed manually by Medicare. This again slows the process and increases the probability of making a second error. Finally, this volume of rejections causes significant confusion and unpredictability within the system. Reducing the confusion and improving the predictability of payment and cash flow could only enhance our financial stability.

Project Team

The first step to quality improvement involved developing an interdisciplinary project team with representation and support from high levels of both the administration and the medical staff of the institution. The team was composed of representatives from all disciplines that affect the accuracy and timeliness of billing of Medicare inpatient services. Most notably, this included representatives from the medical staff; patient care services including admitting, medical records, and utilization management; financial services; and management information services.

Two "project co-owners" who were at high levels of the organization and had administrative responsibility for many of the areas critically involved in the billing process were chosen to coordinate quality improvement efforts.

Identifying Causes of Rejects and Delays

Data quantifying various facets of the problem were presented to the project team. Very early in the investigation, it became clear that the chosen problem involved a multitude of departments. A flow diagram was developed and presented to demonstrate the complex interrelationships of the activities that feed into the final billing process. Together, the data and the flow diagram identified specific areas as targets for improvement.

Billing Inaccuracies

Based on the one-month sample of November 1987, MGH was receiving an average of 160 Medicare inpatient claim rejections per month. This compared to the actual billed claims of approximately 850–900 per month, excluding rebilled claims. On inspection, three reasons for rejections appeared most frequently. Missing or invalid health insurance claim numbers (HIC numbers) accounted for 20 percent of the sampled rejected claims. Nearly 12 percent were rejected because Medicare was billed as the primary payer when Medicare was actually the secondary payer (MSP). Finally, 10 percent of the rejections were

Exhibit C.7. Common Reasons for Rejection, 10/29/87–11/20/87
(Massachusetts General Hospital Project).

Reasons for Rejection	No. of Claims	Percent of Claims
Invalid/Missing HIC No.	32	20.0
Medicare Secondary Payer (MSP)	19	11.9
Excess Ancillary Lines	13	8.1
Covered/Noncovered Days	15	9.4
Invalid MD ID No.	10	6.2
Invalid Total Charges	9	5.6
ICD-9-CM Dx Code	8	5.0
LOA/No Match	7	4.4
FY Split	7	4.4
Other	40	25.0
TOTAL	160	100%

Total billed in this time period = 850

Source: Rejection notification, November 1987.

automatically rejected by Medicare's electronic editing system due to excess ancillary lines on the claim. Exhibit C.7 shows a listing of those and other most commonly occurring reasons for rejections sampled in November 1987.

Inspection of the rejected claims also demonstrated that a disproportionate share of the "hard copy" claims (billed manually, rather than via electronic tape) were being rejected. While only 20 percent of all Medicare claims are billed manually, nearly 50 percent of the Medicare rejections were hard copy claims. This correlation of rejections with manually billed claims was apparent across nearly all reasons for rejections (see Exhibits C.8 and C.9). In addition, inspection of rejected claims demonstrated that nearly 60 percent of the rejections were related to emergency admissions (see Exhibits C.10 and C.11).

Billing Delays

Data indicated that 100 percent of the claims delayed longer than the eight-day target could be attributed to delays in ICD-9 CM coding of the medical record, a requirement for Medicare billing. Coding could commence only after a medi-

Exhibit C.8. Rejections—Hardcopy Versus Electronic Tape,
November 1987 (Baseline) (Massachusetts General Hospital Project).

Reason	Hardcopy		Tape		Total	
	#	%	#	%	#	%
HIC	15	46.9	17	53.1	32	100
MSP	0	0.0	19	100.0	19	100
Excess Ancillary Lines	0	0.0	13	100.0	13	100
Coverage/Noncoverage	12	80.0	3	20.0	15	100
Physican ID	5	50.0	5	50.0	10	100
Invalid Total Charges	9	100.0	0	0.0	9	100
Dx Code	6	75.0	2	25.0	8	100
LOA Days/No Match	3	42.9	4	57.1	7	100
FY Split	7	100.0	0	0.0	7	100
Other/Miscellaneous	22	55.0	18	45.0	40	100
TOTAL	79	49.4%	81	50.6%	160	100%

Source: Medicare Claim Rejection Notifications, 11/1/87–11/31/87.

Exhibit C.9. Rejections: Hard Copy Versus Tape,
November 1987 (Baseline) (Massachusetts General Hospital Project).

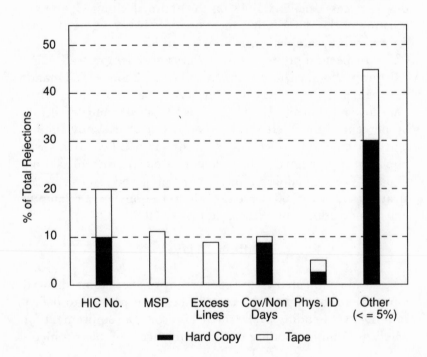

Exhibit C.10. Rejections: Emergency Versus Elective Admissions, November 1987 (Baseline) (Massachusetts General Hospital Project).

Reason	Emergency		Elective		Total	
	#	%	#	%	#	%
HIC	25	78.1%	7	21.9%	32	100.0%
MSP	9	47.4%	10	52.6%	19	100.0%
Excess Ancillary Lines	7	53.8%	6	46.2%	13	100.0%
Coverage/Noncoverage	7	46.7%	8	53.3%	15	100.0%
Physician ID	6	60.0%	4	40.0%	10	100.0%
Invalid Total Charges	4	44.4%	5	55.6%	9	100.0%
Dx Code	6	75.0%	2	25.0%	8	100.0%
LOA Days/No Match	3	42.9%	4	57.1%	7	100.0%
FY Split	3	42.9%	4	57.1%	7	100.0%
Other/Miscellaneous	24	60.0%	16	40.0%	40	100.0%
TOTAL	94	58.8%	66	41.2%	160	100.0%

Source: Medicare Claim Rejection Notifications, 11/1/87–11/31/87.

Exhibit C.11. Rejections: Emergency Versus Elective, November 1987 (Baseline) (Massachusetts General Hospital Project).

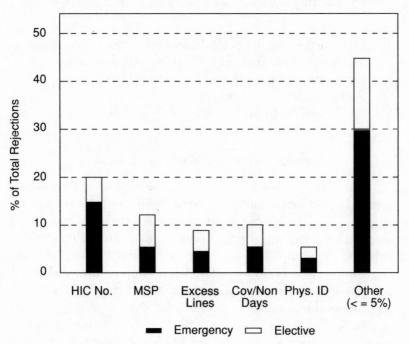

cal record had been attested. Medicare requires that the responsible physician document all diagnoses and procedures associated
with the admission and sign a statement "attesting" to the verac-
ity of this information. Thus, many billing delays may have been
primarily due to lack of physician attestation and, in turn, lack
of coding. In any case, it became clear that reducing the delays
in billing would require a reexamination of the delays in the
medical records function of coding and the physician function
of attestation.

At this point, a very detailed flow diagram of activities
impacting the billing process was developed. A more general
flow chart ("high-level") is included as Exhibit C.12. Both the
process of developing the flow diagram and the diagram itself
enhanced each department's understanding of internal customer-
supplier relationships — that is, how one area affects the next in
the production of a "clean bill." The flow diagram clearly identified areas where the process can falter and where one activity's
output does not match the next activity's requirements.

From this exercise, five goals were developed:

1. Improve the accuracy of HIC number information at admission.
2. Improve the accuracy of MSP information at admission.
3. Eliminate rejections due to "excess anxillary lines."
4. Reduce hard copy claim errors.
5. Reexamine the attestation and coding functions to reduce delays.

Improvement and Associated Results

Given the causes of claim rejections and billing delays,
several departments that have responsibility for these issues were
targeted for quality improvements. They included admitting,
medical records, and inpatient accounting. Improvements involved greater emphasis on: obtaining accurate HIC number and
MSP information upon admission; developing an MGH computerized edit to identify excess ancillary charges, which must
be processed manually; increased employee education regarding quality hard copy claim generation; and restructuring the coding and attestation functions within the medical records department.

Exhibit C.12. Medicare Inpatient Billing Process:
High-Level Flow Diagram (Massachusetts General Hospital Project).

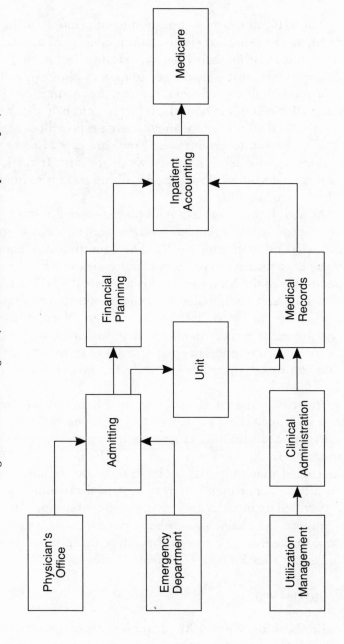

HIC Number Information

The HIC number is easily found imprinted on the patient's Medicare card. For elective admissions, patients are told ahead of time to bring their Medicare card to the hospital. The admitting coordinator is instructed to make a photocopy of the card for the billing record when the patient is admitted. If no card is available at admission, the billing record is "red-tagged." The patient is then visited by an admitting representative, and the family is asked to produce the Medicare card. Emergency admissions are also asked for their Medicare card. If available, the card is photocopied; if not, the admitting sheet is red-tagged and the patient is visited.

Although this process was in place before the study, the quality improvement project has brought more importance to the value of HIC number information. The admitting and financial planning departments have become more aware of how crucial the photocopy of the Medicare card is to verify the HIC number information, and compliance with the photocopying requirement when the card is available has improved. Needless to say, many patients, especially in emergency situations, forget their Medicare card. It remains the policy to admit these patients and then do as much as possible to verify the HIC number.

Results.   The focus on obtaining the correct HIC number has improved the accuracy of this front-end information. Nevertheless, the admitting process continues to suffer from task redundancy. In the current process, the HIC number information is copied manually first by three separate sections within the admitting department, then by financial planning, and is finally verified by inpatient accounting before billing. Through this cumbersome chain, the probability of human error is increased. In the future, a reorganization of this process may be the only way to achieve zero defects in this area.

MSP Information

Establishing whether Medicare is the primary or secondary payer for a particular patient requires knowledge of the various rules that dictate this determination. Currently, an "MSP form" has been designed by the inpatient accounting department to assist admitting coordinators in determining if Medicare is the secondary or primary payer. At this time, use of the form by admitting coordinators is irregular, and the form is almost never used for emergency patients. Furthermore, much of the information on the form is duplicated elsewhere.

While better compliance in using the form at admission may yield slight improvements in MSP information, the future goal will be to establish better communication channels between Medicare billing specialists and admitting coordinators. Through enhanced communication, both groups may develop greater consensus regarding (1) what information is absolutely required in order to assign the payer and (2) who will be responsible for getting which pieces of information.

"Excess Ancillary Lines" Rejections

This rejection involves a front-end edit by Medicare, in which tape claims are automatically rejected because the claims contain too many ancillary charge lines. Such claims must be billed manually. Previously, our system was not properly flagging such claims to alert our billing department to generate a hard copy claim. Once the problem was identified, the appropriate edit was installed to prevent such electronic tape errors.

Results. The rejection rate due to excess ancillary lines has since dropped from twenty-six rejects in October 1987 to an average of six rejects per month in 1988. In addition, other system edits have been developed to further prevent electronic tape errors.

The statistics used to analyze these results were implemented and measured consistently from October 1987 to April 1988. Significant improvement was exhibited over this seven-month period, and the initial issue of Medicare rejections has for the most part been addressed

As our quality team will testify, the only effective improvement process is one that allows its measurement tools to change with evolving external requirements. Since April 1988, our program has adopted new tools, the results of which are not comparable to results gathered during the initial six months shown here. We are confident that our efforts did, however, address the initial goal of reducing our rejections and improving our process.

Hard Copy Claim Errors

Prior to this study, the major emphasis in the manual billing area of inpatient accounting had been volume output. In order to reduce a large and growing accounts receivable balance, first priority was given to getting the claims out the door. As a result of this volume emphasis compounded by staffing vacancies and turnover, the accuracy of the claims suffered. Human error was unavoidable and persistent.

In December 1987 priority was shifted from emphasizing *volume* to emphasizing *quality*. Errors were brought to the attention of individual billers. In addition, all Medicare billers participated in training and educational sessions to improve bill-generation techniques.

Results.   In time, human errors including miscalculated charges, transposed HIC numbers, and blank fields on the claims were reduced. The result has been a marked decline in the rejection of hard copy claims. MGH received seventy-seven rejections of hard copy claims in November 1987. This number dropped to sixty-six in December, fifty in January 1988, and less than thirty for February, March, and April.

Naturally, the added emphasis on quality and accuracy reduced the output of claims in this area. Initially, the accounts receivable balance may show slight increases. Nevertheless, this added short-term cost should be offset by the long-term benefit of a reduced rate of rejections, less processing and rebilling effort, and better cash flow based on more accurate billing.

Attestation and Coding Functions

As the November 1987 data had shown, the critical functions that were most commonly delaying billing were the attestation and the medical record coding function. Based on this understanding, major process changes were initiated as of March 1, 1988.

Attestation. To address the issue of timely attestation, which is important not only for billing but also to ensure a completed record, the following system was designed to hasten attestation. Beginning March 8, 1988, whenever a nonattested record was received in the medical records department, rather than delay the coding process, the coders reviewed the record and coded it as they deemed appropriate before sending it back to the physician. In addition, an autogenerated form was sent to the responsible physician listing all coded diagnoses and procedures for his or her review, correction if necessary, and signature.

In this way, attestation was facilitated and valuable time gained in the billing process.

Coding. Finally, and perhaps more crucial, has been the institution's redesign of the medical record coding function. In recent times, coding has taken on new importance. Not only does delayed coding slow the billing process, but inaccurate coding can also increase the number of rejected bills audited by Medicare and by the Massachusetts Peer Review Organization.

Although coding is an administrative responsibility delegated to the medical records department, it is intimately related to physician behavior and physician documentation. As a result of the tender balance between needing to gather and code medical information quickly yet interpret this information accurately and optimally, the function is a sophisticated one.

For these reasons, MGH has reorganized the coding function into its own department called "Coding and DRG Analysis," which has set specific standards for coding and will implement systems of measurement so that the institution can monitor both the effectiveness and efficiency of this complicated function.

Overall Results

Rejects in all categories decreased dramatically as a result of the team's intervention (see Exhibit C.13). HIC number rejects were reduced 45 percent from the November 1987 baseline

Exhibit C.13. Reasons for Rejection Notifications for the Period
November 1987 to April 1988 (Massachusetts General Hospital Project).

Month	Invalid or Missing HIC No.	Excess Ancillary Lines	Medicare Secondary Payer
October		26	
November	32	13	19
December	18	3	12
January	15	7	12
February	23	4	8
March	19	8	53
April	17	7	6

to April 1988. Excess ancillary charge rejects were reduced 73
percent and MSP rejects 75 percent. Also, the number of incomplete medical records decreased 30 percent from January
1988 to March 1988 (see Exhibit C.14).

Improved Accuracy

To measure the overall accuracy of the billing process,
the number of claim rejections received per month was monitored as improvements in the process were implemented. As
Exhibit C.15 shows, the number of monthly rejections has decreased from a high of 160 in November to 76 in April 1988.

With increased concentration on the quality of each claim,
the quantity of bills generated has decreased somewhat. This
trend will be carefully monitored to fully understand its implications. Over this same period of time, HIC number rejections
have decreased from thirty-two to seventeen. MSP rejections
have declined from nineteen to six. Excess ancillary line rejects
have dropped from twenty-six in October 1987 to seven in April
1988. Finally, the number of hard copy rejects has dropped from
seventy-nine to seventeen in April 1988.

Improved Medical Record Documentation

Since March 1, 1988, when the new attestation form and
process were initiated, the number of incomplete medical records

Exhibit C.14. Incomplete Medical Records, January 1988–April 1988
(Massachusetts General Hospital Project).

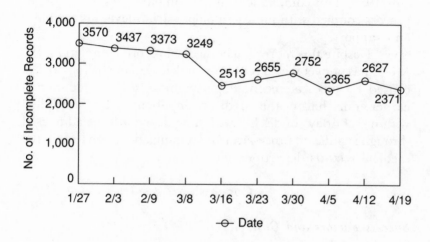

Exhibit C.15. Rejections: Total and Hard Copy,
November 1987–April 1988
(Massachusetts General Hospital Project).

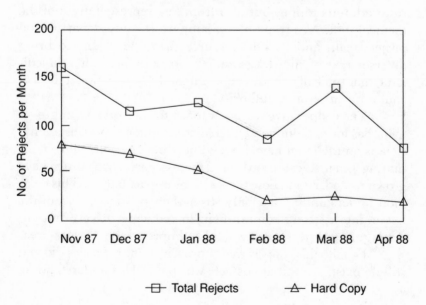

on any one day has significantly declined. Exhibit C.14 illustrates this trend from over 3,500 incomplete records in January 1988 to an average of about 2,200 incomplete records through July 1989. This compliance has been in part a result of a better process coupled with more senior physician-level involvement and support.

Despite this more timely medical record completion, the MGH has not yet seen a reduction in delays to the billing process caused by medical record department issues. As mentioned earlier, only half of the Medicare inpatient claims are billed within eight days of discharge. These delays will be addressed through significant procedural and organizational reviews in the medical records department.

Conclusion

Success Factors and Obstacles

Without question, the most instrumental factor to the success in reducing billing inaccuracies and analyzing billing delays has been the commitment from high levels of the organization to solve the problem. This commitment has come not only from administration, but also from key representatives of the medical staff. As a result of this support, the interdepartmental project team and its staff resources have been able to bring diverse areas of knowledge and expertise to focus on a difficult issue that typically crosses departmental and functional lines of communication and authority.

The cooperative team approach toward quality improvement has forged common understanding among specialists. Physicians on the team have learned how their actions impact admitting and medical records, and these departments in turn have grown to understand how their actions impact billing. This common understanding has only strengthened what was from the beginning a strong commitment to reducing defects and encouraging progress toward quality improvement in this area.

Despite this cooperative approach, some obstacles did and still do exist. An initial obstacle was the lack of understanding within separate departments about the activities, requirements, and priorities of the next step in the process. Concomitant with this lack of understanding is the ongoing lack of common measurements or indicators of quality within and between departments. In-house data describing the billing process including compliance to requirements are not regularly collected or analyzed. Furthermore, due to delays in rejection notification from Medicare, it remains difficult to provide timely and adequate feedback regarding performance on areas for improvement.

A second obstacle is the challenge of communicating with and encouraging compliance regarding medical documentation requirements from the sizable physician staff. As the flow diagram (Exhibit C.12) demonstrates, physicians greatly influence the ability to generate accurate and timely bills. The full support and commitment of the highest levels of the administrative and physician leadership will be necessary to meet this challenge.

Finally, MGH, like other health care providers, faces the obstacle of an ever-changing regulatory environment that determines Medicare benefit coverage, billing specifications, and reimbursement methods. Medicare requirements for a "clean bill" can change without warning, and the method of rejection notification can be inconsistent and unpredictable. Given these issues, even a high-quality process of billing can quickly become outdated and undesirable. Without an ongoing and adaptive quest for improvement, this environmental obstacle will clearly hinder any success in maintaining the level of quality to which the institution has committed.

Next Steps

Much improvement is still possible. Primary to this continued improvement must be improved communication among admitting, financial planning, and inpatient accounting. At this point, several tasks are duplicated by the three areas without clear accountability given to any one area. The goal of this communication can be to establish mutual understanding regarding what information is critical and who is responsible for assuring the quality of that information.

A second objective is to better understand the elevated rejection rate for claims of patients admitted through the emergency department. Clearly, these patients are not only the most likely to forget their Medicare cards but also the most difficult to interview for financial information. Management in this area is preparing to fully implement the hospital's credit and collection policy as it relates to emergency services and a professional billing scheme. These activities involve a significant focus and review of the current registration process in the emergency department, which should ultimately improve the information collected in terms of both completeness and quality. This in turn should lead to fewer rejected claims.

A third goal for the future is to establish more rigorous guidelines for the area of medical record coding. Is there a way to streamline the process? Can we educate physicians to facilitate rather than impede the attestation and coding process? Can we be not only effective but also efficient in that area?

Most crucial to the success of each of these future goals will be the development of information systems that can provide accessible and regular measurement data. What use are standards if one cannot tell whether the standard is being achieved or not? Finally, the MGH must begin to design incentives for compliance to the standards set. Why should an admitting coordinator be accurate in collecting the HIC number if the cost of inaccuracy is borne by some area further downstream? The incentive will need to be relevant, not just to the billing area, but to the many clinical and administrative departments that impact the final bill for Medicare inpatient services.

Lessons for Health Care Quality

One of the most striking insights gained from this project has been an appreciation of the complexity of problems that span multiple departmental areas. The billing process was chosen as a problem that seemed somewhat "contained" or at least administratively "controllable." Nevertheless, investigation of the root causes of the problem has demonstrated that many areas impact this process. Indeed, what at first seemed to be an administrative problem is intricately related to the medical staff and their behavior. Bringing quality to this arena in which no single department has authority or control over the final product has forced the MGH to understand and adapt to the complexity of the institution's organizational structure.

The project showed how severe can be the cost of rework and how much light can be shed by cross-functional teams on complex processes that no single individual or department fully understood.

In addition to revealing the internal complexity of the institution, the project has demonstrated the challenges of managing within a dynamic external environment. Along with the quality improvement initiatives, several outside forces have impacted the billing process. As in any social science research, it is difficult to specify cause-and-effect relationships without a controlled environment. Nevertheless, the MGH has experienced improvements. Only time will tell whether these initiatives can be sustained and even enhanced as the environment continues to change.

Undoubtedly, the data-collection and analysis activities have done much to enhance interdepartmental understanding of billing defects and each area's responsibility to prevent defects. The specific techniques of problem identification, flowcharting, and cause analysis aided our progress. These could not have come into play without commitment from high-level administration and medical staff. Such commitment fostered an increased focus of resources on a problem with the common goal of quality improvement.

Park Nicollet Medical Center: Improving Patient Access*

Park Nicollet Medical Center, Minneapolis

Regular patients sometimes drop out of the finest of medical centers. Potential patients make appointments and never show up. Others never get through on the phone. They all go somewhere else, where they are likely to stay for many years unless and until they are dissatisfied.

Patients phone doctors for a variety of reasons. They may want to know the results of tests, answers to questions about a prescribed medicine, advice about a new problem, or evaluation in the office. Whatever the reason, the patient who calls and gets a busy signal is going to be dissatisfied, and care may be compromised.

Project Selection

At the Park Nicollet Medical Center, when we surveyed over 7,000 patients, a preliminary list of twenty-three likely causes of dissatisfaction was put into questionnaire form. Exhibit C.16 is a Pareto diagram showing the frequency with which each source of dissatisfaction was cited.

Of the twenty-three potential causes surveyed, six were found not to be contributors; thus the exhibit shows only seventeen. Of the contributors, the one that the team expected to show up as the leading cause of dissatisfaction (waiting room time) generated fewer responses than two other contributors. The ranking of "telephone access" (that is, difficulty getting through to physician or having to wait long) as the leading cause of

*By James L. Reinertsen, M.D., President and Chief Executive Officer Park Nicollet Medical Center; David Bush, Ph.D., Department of Psychology, Villanova University; Robert S. Schimmel, Director of Consulting Services, Park Nicollet Medical Center; John A. Haugen, M.D., Chairman, Department of Family Practice; Michele S. Barton, R.N., Family Practice, Park Nicollet Medical Center; Kathi L. Evenson, R.N., Family Practice, Park Nicollet Medical Center; John R. Kasminski, M.D., Family Practice, Park Nicollet Medical Center.

dissatisfaction was unexpected, and its dominance among the "vital few" led the team to undertake analyses of causes contributing to the telephone access problem itself.

Telephone access was by far the leading cause of patient dissatisfaction. Moreover, this problem was prominent in all departments and sites. The clinic's administrative team was aware of the phone problem, but had been unable to come up with solutions (short of simply adding expensive capacity). Therefore, telephone access seemed to be a good problem with which to test the application of "industrial" quality management techniques.

Our surveys also showed that many of the departments with telephone access problems also seemed to have "acute appointment" access problems. In the course of this project, we hoped to gain some insight into the relationship, if any, between telephone access and acute appointment access.

Project Team

The project team consisted of:

1. The family practice section of the main office of Park Nicollet Medical Center — five family practitioners, six hall nurses, two medical information (MI) nurses, four receptionists, led by Kathi Evenson, R.N., and Michele Barton, R.N.
2. A central administrative support and analysis group consisting of Robert Schimmel, Director of Consulting Services, and James Reinertsen, M.D., President and Chief Executive Officer.
3. Consultant support and analysis by David Bush, Ph.D., Department of Psychology, Villanova University.

The idea of the project, general goals, and background information was presented to the family practice department (first physicians, then all) in two meetings in the fall of 1987. Basic information on industrial quality management techniques was shared, but formal teaching of statistical methods to all participants was not accomplished. The family practice department

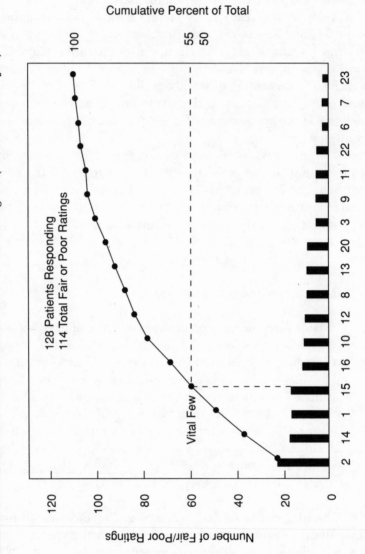

Exhibit C.16. Reasons for Patient Dissatisfaction: A Pareto Diagram (Park Nicollet Project).

Exhibit C.16. Reasons for Patient Dissatisfaction: A Pareto Diagram (Park Nicollet Project), Cont'd.

1. Ease of getting appointment
2. Ability to get through on phone
3. Attitude of phone receptionist
4. Attitude of clinic receptionist
5. Attitude of nurses
6. Willingness of staff to answer questions
7. Cleanliness of clinic
8. Ease of getting around in clinic
9. Attitude of lab personnel
10. Timely response to phone calls
11. Timely prescription refills
12. Billing process

13. Response to complaints
14. Communication about new services
15. Waiting time in reception area
16. Waiting time in examination room
17. Friendliness of doctor
18. Competence of doctor
19. Responsiveness of doctor
20. Amount of time spent with doctor
21. Concern shown by doctor
22. Information given you about diagnosis
23. Overall satisfaction

took day-to-day responsibility for the project, with a small intra-departmental steering group guiding decisions. Central administrative support was used to clear obstacles, such as obtaining CRT access and permission to add a medical information nurse, and to perform phone data abstraction and analysis.

Identifying Causes of Poor Access

The entire process of obtaining medical information and/or an appointment by telephone was thoroughly documented and represented in a process flow diagram (Exhibit C.17). This and the accompanying tallies of phone traffic types and volumes were extremely helpful in describing the elements of the phone access problem. The flow diagram demonstrated how complex our phone information and appointment system is.

Receptionists and nurses were asked to record the types and volumes of calls and their disposition at various points in the flow diagram, for a two-week period, sampling the busiest hours of the morning and afternoon.

The tally of phone traffic types demonstrated a surprising fact — that 75 percent of patients calling in to the doctor's office for an appointment believed that their problem required that they be seen within twenty-four hours. Since only 10 or 15 percent of each day's schedule was reserved for such patients, the resulting mismatch of patients' perceptions and doctors' schedules needed to be addressed as well.

Cause-and-effect diagrams allowed all members of the family practice department — receptionists, nurses, physicians, and managers — to see the many dimensions of the telephone problem (see Exhibit C.18). Priorities were difficult to establish, however.

Control charts proved to be more useful. The telephone system in place at Park Nicollet provided excellent data on call volumes, calls abandoned, and average time to answer a call. These reports were reformatted into control charts such as Exhibit C.19.

Initially the charts were developed and displayed for two-week blocks, which resulted in a "blurring" of a good deal of useful detail. After review of the day-to-day and hour-to-hour variation in phone access, we revised the chart format to reflect hourly statistics. The hourly control chart proved to be a much more useful analytical management tool. For example, Exhibit C.19 pointed out the dramatic effect on phone access for the one hour that two receptionists were called away for important training meetings. (Following this observation, we changed the training policy immediately to avoid taking receptionists away from their positions during business hours.)

During a ten-day period in December, we gathered baseline data on "average time to answer" and "percent abandoned calls" (patient hung up before anyone answered). After this initial data gathering was completed, it became apparent that the telephone access problem was most severe at the level of the medical information (MI) nurse in the flow diagram. During the ten days in December, the average time to answer the MI nurse phone was one to one and a half minutes, whereas the average time to answer the receptionist phone was fifteen seconds.

We therefore chose to focus most of our effort on the MI nurse problem. In January, we began to track the "average time to answer" (AvTAn) and "abandoned call percentage" (AbCP) for the MI nurses and receptionists and began to report the two-week average AvTAn and AbCP to the department within a few days of the end of each period (Exhibit C.20).

Initial Improvements

The department initiated a series of uncontrolled experiments to attempt to improve the MI nurses' AvTAn and AbCP. The initial actions were based on the cause-and-effect diagram and included:

1. Empowering the MI nurse to put patients into a physician's "acute care time" without need for physician authorization.
2. Increasing the available "acute care time" of two of the five physicians by 10 percent.

The results of those actions alone were disappointing. We therefore went back to the data and reviewed it, not in two-week

Exhibit C.17. Same-Day Medical Need Family Practice, Park Campus Office: A Process Flow Diagram (Park Nicollet Project).

Exhibit C.17. Same-Day Medical Need Family Practice, Park Campus Office:
A Process Flow Diagram (Park Nicollet Project), Cont'd.

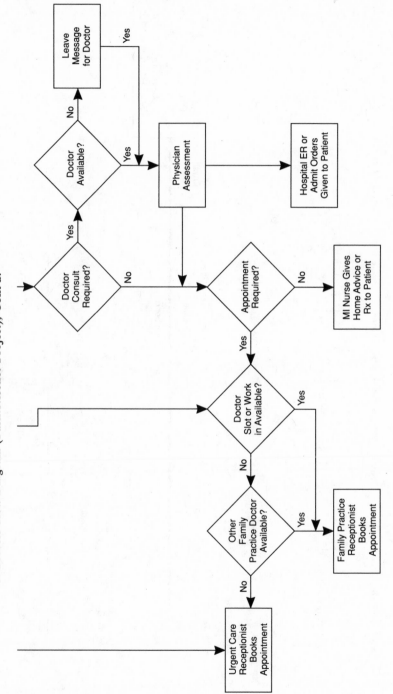

Exhibit C.18. Reasons Contributing to Telephone Access Problems: A Cause-and-Effect Diagram (Park Nicollet Project).

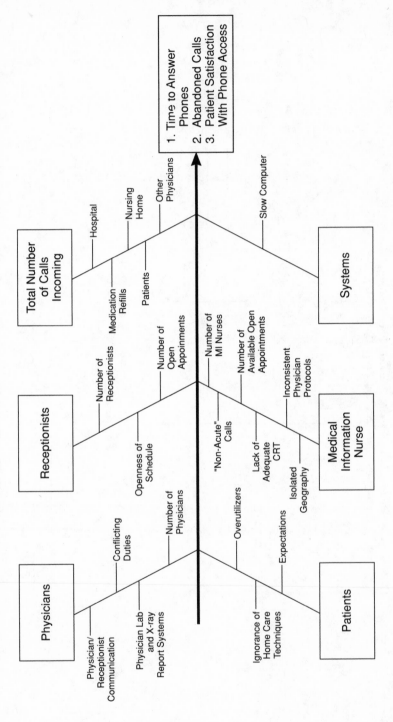

blocks but *hour-by-hour* (Exhibit C.22). This clearly showed that the worst problem was from 8:00 to 11:00 A.M.

We decided to try a two-week experiment during which we would deal with this additional insight, along with previously unaddressed "causes" on the cause-effect diagram. Accordingly, we prepared to do an hour-by-hour report of phone access for two weeks and initiated the following changes during that test period:

1. An additional MI nurse was brought in from 8:00 A.M. to 1:00 P.M.
2. The "regular" MI nurse started at 8:00 A.M. rather than 8:30 A.M.
3. Approximately 40 percent of each physician's daily schedule was kept "open."
4. Both the MI nurses *and* the receptionists were empowered to use their best judgment to put any patient with an acute need into the physicians' schedules that day, without the need to obtain the physician's permission.

The effect of this two-week experiment on MI nurse phone access was to reduce the mean AvTAn from 203 to 103 seconds during the last two weeks in April and to narrow the control limits substantially (Exhibit C.22).

There were other initial effects of the experiment, however. Receptionists and MI nurses were delighted with the ease with which they could place patients into schedules. Physicians, on the other hand, observed that many of the patients seen during the experiment were patients who did not need a physician's attention and would not have achieved access to their schedules under the "old" system of appointments. In many cases, these patients had self-limiting conditions that would have gone away before they could have gained access to the physician under the old system.

We documented the extent of this problem, since it did not make sense to have excellent phone and appointment access but to "waste" an expensive resource like a physician's time.

Exhibit C.19. Average Time to Answer Telephones Between 9:00 and 10:00 A.M. (Park Nicollet Project).

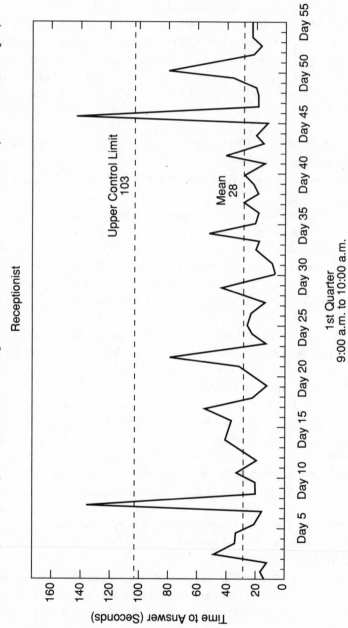
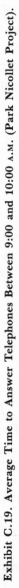

Exhibit C.19. Average Time to Answer Telephones Between 9:00 and 10:00 A.M. (Park Nicollet Project), Cont'd.

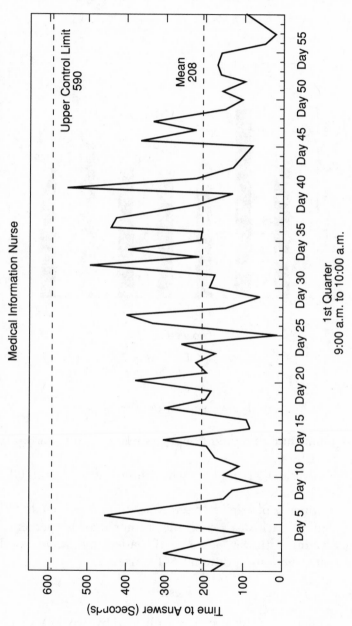

Medical Information Nurse

Exhibit C.20. Time to Answer Telephones and Abandoned Call Rate:
Baseline Period (Park Nicollet Project).

Receptionist: Average Time to Answer

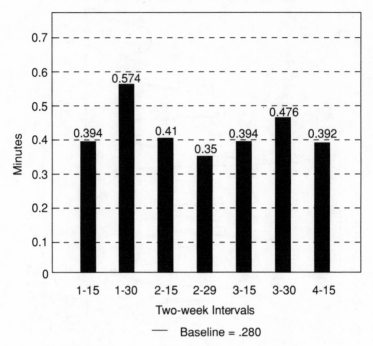

Two-week Intervals

— Baseline = .280

Subsequently, we settled on the following:

1. Continuing the additional MI nurse time from 8:00 A.M. to 1:00 P.M.
2. Giving the MI nurses "scheduling training" on a CRT at their station.
3. Reducing physician "open time" to approximately 20 percent of each day's schedule, rather than 40 percent, and dealing with the "acute need" patient by phone — perhaps with even an additional MI nurse.

Results

Success on this project is indicated by two measures. The principal goal was to reduce AvTAn on the MI nurse line, and

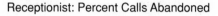

Exhibit C.20. Time to Answer Telephones and Abandoned Call Rate: Baseline Period (Park Nicollet Project), Cont'd.

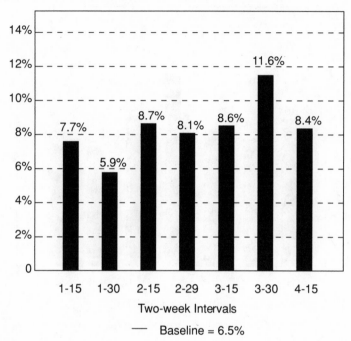

we have reduced it from 208 to 103 seconds. The additional labor cost in order to achieve these gains was approximately $42 per day.

Conclusion

Our experience supports the conclusion that industrial quality management techniques can aid in improving the quality of service in health care. We have not applied these techniques to professional care problems, but plan to do so in the near future.

We have also relearned an age-old lesson, namely, "We don't ever solve problems; we simply choose the problems we want to live with." In our case, we initially made a modest improvement in phone access at the expense of a possible decrease

Exhibit C.20. Time to Answer Telephones and Abandoned Call Rate:
Baseline Period (Park Nicollet Project), Cont'd.

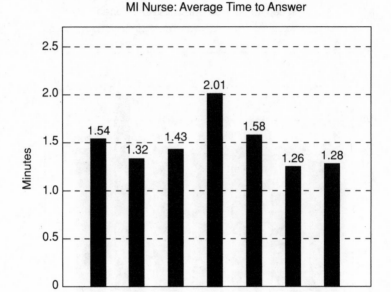

MI Nurse: Average Time to Answer

— Baseline = 1.17

in physician efficiency. We had to address the second problem
while further improving the first.

The final lesson we learned is that our telephone appoint-
ment/information system will require either additional capacity
(for example, more MI nurses, more doctors) or radical redesign
in order for greater gains to be achieved. We are considering
both possibilities, all the while keeping in mind our mission —
the highest quality health care and service possible.

In retrospect, we believe that we could have made more
rapid gains if we had:

- Spent more time educating department members on the
  basic "tools."
- Done a more detailed statistical analysis of our preliminary

Exhibit C.20. Time to Answer Telephones and Abandoned Call Rate:
Baseline Period (Park Nicollet Project), Cont'd.

MI Nurse: Percent Calls Abandoned

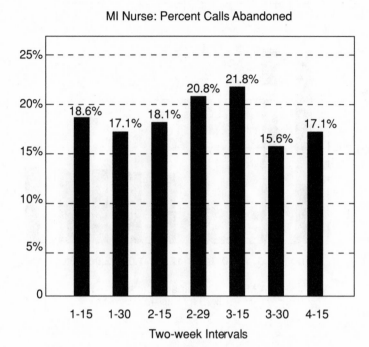

Two-week Intervals

— Baseline = 13.5%

data; we might have appreciated the importance of an hour-by-hour control chart early on. (This insight was eventually gained by involving Dr. Bush in the project more deeply. We believe we should have "asked him in" earlier and in greater depth.)

• Taken department time to meet every week or two to review all statistics; a smaller steering group did so, but communication with the larger department was perhaps not as detailed as it could have been.

• Recognized the gap between the family practitioners' ideal practice concept (that is, scheduled appointments, preventive care, and so on) and what their patients appear to want (that is, lots of acute care appointment access or "urgent care").

Exhibit C.21. Average Time for Medical Information Nurse to Answer
Telephones, Stratified by Hour of the Day (Park Nicollet Project).

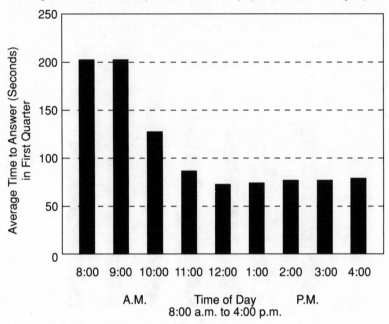

Addendum

Park Nicollet is now applying the principles of continuous quality improvement systemwide, with the consulting support of the Total Quality Management team from the 3M Company. 3M has successfully implemented these principles for years
and has had some success "exporting" their expertise to hospitals. The continuous quality improvement process is central to
our strategy — to be perceived the unquestioned leader in quality of care and service in our marketplace.

Exhibit C.22. Average Time for Medical Information Nurse to Answer Telephones Between 9:00 and 10:00 A.M. (Park Nicollet Project).

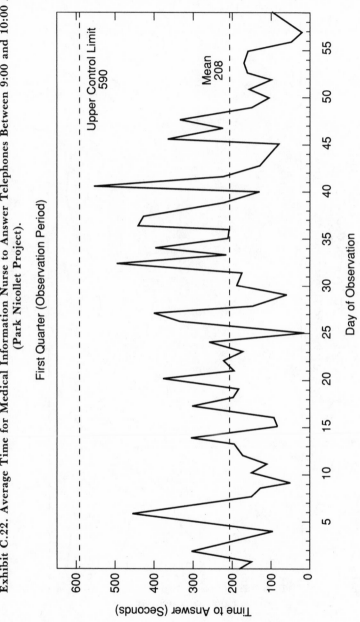

Exhibit C.22. Average Time for Medical Information Nurse to Answer Telephones Between 9:00 and 10:00 A.M. (Park Nicollet Project), Cont'd.

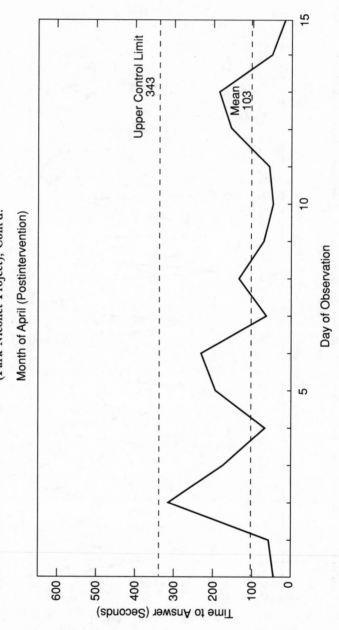

Month of April (Postintervention)

Resource D:
Key Readings in
Quality Improvement

The following is a short, representative list of useful further readings on quality management. With more space, we could have named many more excellent books, articles, and videotapes that can help deepen expertise in the field. Those who want a wider listing can contact the American Society for Quality Control (ASQC), at 310 West Wisconsin Avenue, Milwaukee, WI 53203 (1-800-952-6587), to obtain ASQC's excellent Quality Press Publications Catalogue. Those who join ASQC also receive a monthly magazine, *Quality Progress,* containing helpful review articles on quality management theory, methods, and applications.

AT&T. *Statistical Quality Control Handbook.* Indianapolis, Ind.: AT&T, 1956.

A classic manual of statistical process control that includes clear instructions for creating and using control charts. This book was developed originally for use in training managers, supervisors, engineers, and other employees at the Western Electric Company.

Berwick, D.M. "Continuous Improvement as an Ideal in Health Care." *New England Journal of Medicine,* 1989, *320,* 53–56.

Explores the potential usefulness of continuous improvement methods in health care, and compares them with current methods of surveillance and quality assurance.

Camp, R. C. *Benchmarking: The Search for Industry Best Practices that Lead to Superior Performance.* Milwaukee, Wis.: ASQC Press, 1989.

Benchmarking is a formal method of identifying and studying better processes and superior products. This is a comprehensive description of the method, which may have wide implications for health care organizations.

Crosby, P. B. *Quality Is Free.* New York: New American Library, 1979.

A widely read and influential book describing the benefits of "doing things right the first time" and setting out a fourteen-step management plan for getting there.

Deming, W. E. *Out of the Crisis.* Cambridge, Mass.: MIT-CAES, 1986.

The major book by one of the leading figures in the quality movement. Contains extended anecdotes and examples illustrating Deming's theory in action.

Feigenbaum, A. V. *Total Quality Control.* New York: McGraw-Hill, 1983.

A practical description of planning, deploying, maintaining, and controlling an effective, companywide quality program. This is an important book that has had an international impact.

Garvin, D. A. *Managing Quality: The Strategic and Competitive Edge.* New York: Free Press, 1988.

A highly readable explanation of how quality management and corporate strategy can and should be linked in a healthy corporation. Garvin makes use of extended examples of breakthrough performance in manufacturing and illustrates practices associated with excellence.

Imai, M. *Kaizen: The Key to Japan's Competitive Success.* New York: Random House, 1986.

An orderly presentation of Japanese quality improvement approaches and the theory of continuous improvement. Describes sixteen specific management practices that can move an organization toward gradual, unending improvement.

Ishikawa, K. *What Is Total Quality Control?* Englewood Cliffs, N.J.: Prentice-Hall, 1985.

One of the most widely used manuals of statistical quality control and quality improvement methods in Japan. Presents the tools at a practical level.

Juran, J. M. *Managerial Breakthrough.* New York: McGraw-Hill, 1964.

A major work setting out the logical basis for performance breakthroughs that can be achieved with quality improvement methods, and the breakthroughs in attitude, organization, knowledge, and culture that must be achieved en route.

Juran, J. M. (ed.). *Juran's Quality Control Handbook.* (4th ed.) New York: McGraw-Hill, 1988.

A massive volume summarizing the major ideas in quality planning, quality improvement, and quality control. An excellent reference book, chapters from which can also be used in training in both technical and organizational areas of quality management.

Juran, J. M. *Juran on Leadership for Quality.* New York: Free Press, 1989.

An executive handbook for quality management that describes the role of upper management in making quality happen.

King, B. *Better Decisions in Half the Time: Implementing Quality Function Deployment in America.* Methuen, Mass.: Goal/QPC, 1989.

A complete, somewhat technical overview of quality function deployment as an approach to planning and design.

McGregor, D. *The Human Side of Enterprise.* New York: McGraw-Hill, 1960.

McGregor's research and this classic book describing the "Theory X" and "Theory Y" approaches to management made a major contribution to the organization development aspects of quality management theory.

Mizuno, S. *Company-Wide Total Quality Control.* Tokyo: Asian Productivity Organization, 1987.

An extended prescription for organizationwide quality control. This book contains a number of useful checklists of activities and methods; it will appeal to those who desire a highly structured exposition of the attributes of the quality-minded organization.

Plsek, P. E., Onnias, A., and Early, J. F. *Quality Improvement Tools.* Wilton, Conn.: Juran Institute, Inc., 1989.

A straightforward introduction to ten of the basic tools for quality improvement. Useful as instructional materials for teams and leaders.

Reich, R. B. "Entrepreneurship Reconsidered: The Team as Hero." *Harvard Business Review,* 1987, *65,* 77–83.

A brief article exploring how compensation, reward, and recognition systems might better encourage the sort of teamwork demanded in quality improvement.

Scherkenbach, W. W. *The Deming Route to Quality and Productivity.* Rockville, Md.: Mercury Press, 1986.

A short volume with a succinct summary of Deming's basic model of quality management by the expert who helped Ford Motor Company change its ways.

Scholtes, P. R. *The Team Handbook.* Madison, Wis.: Joiner Associates, 1988.

One of the best available manuals for team activity in quality improvement. Takes the reader step-by-step through the organizing, training, leadership, and process improvement work of teams, and clearly explains the underlying managerial and statistical principles.

Tufte, E. R. *The Visual Display of Quantitative Information.* Cheshire, Conn.: Graphics Press, 1983.

A delightful exploration of how graphic tools of all sorts can help tap and display information. Explains the properties of both good charts and bad ones.

Wadsworth, H. M., Jr., Stephens, K. S., and Godfrey, A. B. *Modern Methods for Quality Control and Improvement.* New York: Wiley, 1986.

A comprehensive textbook emphasizing graphical methods and statistical tools for process control and improvement, with brief excursions into the relevant statistical theory.

Walton, M. *The Deming Management Method.* New York: Putnam, 1986.

A highly readable summary of Deming's theories and his "Fourteen Points" on proper management methods. This is one of the best available introductory readings on this approach to quality improvement.

Index